Volume Two: Materia Medica of Homeopathic Gemstones

Dr Víctor Denis Purcell and Victor Denis Purcell

Published by Dr Víctor Denis Purcell, 2024.

While every precaution has been taken in the preparation of this book, the publisher assumes no responsibility for errors or omissions, or for damages resulting from the use of the information contained herein.

VOLUME TWO: MATERIA MEDICA OF HOMEOPATHIC GEMSTONES

First edition. July 25, 2024.

ISBN: 979-8227701626

Written by Dr Víctor Denis Purcell and Victor Denis Purcell.

Dedication: Alexander, Tayler , Matt and Marco

Volume Two

Materia Medica of Homeopathic Gemstones

Chapter Listing:

Disclaimer ◈

Please read the following terms and conditions carefully before proceeding.

General Information Purposes Only: The information provided in the following is for general information and entertainment purposes only. All information is provided in good faith; however, the author makes no representation or warranty of any kind, express or implied, regarding the accuracy, adequacy, validity, reliability, availability, or completeness of any information on the following.

Not Medical Advice: The content provided below is not intended to be a substitute for professional medical advice, diagnosis, or treatment. Always seek the advice of your physician or other qualified health providers with any questions you may have regarding a medical condition or health concerns.

No Doctor-Patient Relationship: reading the information below does not constitute establishing a doctor-patient relationship. Any health information communicated is not an endorsement, diagnosis, or treatment regimen.

Professional Assistance: You must not rely on the information below as an alternative to medical advice from your doctor or other professional healthcare providers. If you believe you are experiencing any medical condition, seek immediate medical attention from a licensed healthcare provider.

Risks of Self-Diagnosis: Self-diagnosis can lead to harm, and healthcare professionals must perform diagnosis and treatment.

Limitation of Warranties: The medical information provided is "as is" without any representations or warranties, express or implied. The author makes no representations or warranties concerning the medical report.

Liability: You agree to release the author from all liability and to hold him harmless from any legal claims related to the medical information provided.

Contact a doctor: Do not disregard, avoid, or delay obtaining medical advice from a qualified healthcare provider because of something you may have read in this book or below.

You do understand and agree to the terms of this disclaimer. If you do not agree with these terms, you are not authorized to obtain information from or otherwise proceed.

- **Chapter 1, introduction to homeopathic medicine**

In the realm of medical sciences, where evidence-based practices and biochemical interventions dominate the landscape, there exists a field that takes a markedly different approach: homeopathic medicine. This discipline, rooted in the late 18th century, was pioneered by Samuel Hahnemann, a German physician disillusioned by the prevailing medical practices of his time. Homeopathy is founded on principles that challenge conventional medical paradigms, particularly the notions of dosage, symptom treatment, and the nature of healing itself.

This chapter seeks to provide an in-depth introduction to the foundational principles, history, and philosophy that constitute the backbone of homeopathic medicine. By delving into the core concepts of "similia similibus curentur" (like cures like) and the use of highly diluted remedies, it aims to shed light on how homeopathy stimulates the body's intrinsic healing responses. The journey begins with an exploration of the rich historical roots of homeopathy, from its inception by Hahnemann to the evolution and adaptation of his principles over time. Understanding this historical context is crucial, as it reveals the motivations and insights that drove Hahnemann to develop a system of medicine that emphasized gentle, individualized care over the often harsh and invasive treatments of his era.

Central to this discussion is the Law of Similars, which posits that substances capable of producing symptoms in healthy individuals can be used to treat similar symptoms in the sick. This principle was a radical departure from the conventional medical practices of Hahnemann's time and continues to be a cornerstone of homeopathic practice. Through meticulous experimentation and documentation, Hahnemann developed a comprehensive materia medica that guides homeopaths in matching patient symptoms with appropriate remedies.

Another key aspect of homeopathy covered in this chapter is the process of potentization and succussion, methods developed by Hahnemann to prepare remedies in a way that enhances their healing properties while minimizing toxicity. This process of serial dilution and vigorous shaking, which imprints the "memory" of the original substance onto the diluent, challenges conventional pharmacological beliefs but remains a fundamental practice in homeopathic medicine.

The chapter also delves into the principle of the minimum dose, which emphasizes using the smallest possible amount of a substance to stimulate a healing response. This approach aims to avoid side effects and supports the body's natural healing processes without overwhelming them. It reflects a broader philosophical stance within homeopathy that respects the body's inherent wisdom and capacity for self-healing.

Furthermore, this chapter highlights the individualized approach of homeopathic treatment. Unlike the standardized protocols of conventional medicine, homeopathy tailors its remedies to the unique physical, emotional, and mental symptoms of each patient. This personalized care extends to chronic and complex conditions, emphasizing a holistic view of health that integrates mental, emotional, and physical well-being.

The concept of vital force, or vital energy, is also examined. This vitalist perspective views health as a state of dynamic equilibrium maintained by an intrinsic energy force, which, when imbalanced, leads to disease. Homeopathic remedies aim to restore balance to this vital force, a concept that aligns with various traditional healing systems around the world.

Lastly, the chapter addresses the Doctrine of Drug Proving, a method by which homeopaths determine the effects of remedies through systematic testing on healthy individuals. This empirical approach ensures that the therapeutic application of remedies is grounded in direct human experience, emphasizing the importance of subjective reports as valuable diagnostic tools.

This chapter provides a comprehensive overview of homeopathy's unique approach to medicine, one that emphasizes gentle, individualized care, the use of minimal doses, and a holistic view of health. By understanding these principles and their historical development, readers will gain insight into the distinct nature of homeopathic practice and its enduring relevance in the broader field of healthcare.

- **Main content:**

As we have seen in the above, in this chapter, we delve into the fundamental principles, history, and philosophy underpinning homeopathic medicine. We explore the core concepts of "similia similibus curentur" (like cures like) and the utilization of highly diluted remedies to stimulate the body's intrinsic healing mechanisms. Additionally, we trace the historical origins of homeopathy, from its inception by Samuel Hahnemann to the evolution and development of his principles. This foundational understanding will provide readers with a comprehensive overview of this distinct form of medicine.

The Genesis of Homeopathy: Samuel Hahnemann's Vision

The genesis of homeopathy is rooted in the work of Samuel Hahnemann, an 18th-century German physician. Disenchanted with the medical practices of his time—often characterized by harsh and ineffective treatments—Hahnemann sought a more humane and rational approach to healing. His pursuit led to the principle of "similia similibus curentur" or "like cures like," which became the cornerstone of homeopathic medicine. This principle marked a significant departure from the prevailing medical practices of bloodletting, purging, and the use of toxic substances. Hahnemann envisioned a medical system that supported the body's natural healing tendencies, a concept he found echoed in ancient texts but not rigorously applied in a systematic medical framework.

Hahnemann's early life and education were instrumental in shaping his medical philosophy. Born in 1755 in Meissen, Germany, he exhibited a keen intellect and a passion for learning. He studied medicine at the University of Leipzig and later at the University of Erlangen, where he was awarded his MD. His dissatisfaction with the crude and often harmful medical practices of his time drove him to seek alternatives. His profound knowledge of chemistry, pharmacology, and various languages allowed him to access a broad range of medical texts, further fueling his quest for a better healing system.

The Law of Similars: Understanding "Like Cures Like"

The foundational principle of homeopathy, "like cures like," posits that substances capable of causing disease symptoms in healthy individuals can treat similar symptoms in the sick. Hahnemann's discovery was catalyzed by his observation of the effects of cinchona bark (quinine) in treating malaria, noting that it produced malaria-like symptoms in healthy individuals. This observation led to further experimentation and the formulation of a doctrine suggesting that substances inducing symptoms in healthy individuals could be used to stimulate the body's healing processes. This law signified a profound interconnectedness between humans and nature, which homeopathy seeks to harness.

As Hahnemann continued his experiments, he documented the specific effects of various substances on healthy individuals, a process termed "provings." Volunteers, including Hahnemann himself, would ingest a substance and meticulously record the resulting physical, emotional, and mental symptoms. These observations formed the rudimentary materia medica of homeopathy, guiding the selection of remedies to match a patient's symptom profile.

Hahnemann further refined the preparation of homeopathic remedies through a method known as potentization, which involves systematic dilution and succussion (vigorous shaking) at each dilution step. He proposed that this process not only reduced the toxicity of the substance but also enhanced its therapeutic properties, even when diluted beyond the point of containing any molecules of the original substance. Hahnemann's work with provings extended over many years and involved a wide range of substances, including plants, minerals, and animal products. His dedication to rigorously testing these substances on himself and other volunteers provided a wealth of empirical data that formed the backbone of homeopathic practice.

Individualized treatment is another pivotal element of homeopathy. Unlike the one-size-fits-all approach of conventional medicine, homeopathy emphasizes the uniqueness of each patient's illness experience. Effective treatment requires a thorough understanding of the patient's symptoms, lifestyle, and psychological state, acknowledging the complexity of human health and tailoring remedies to the individual rather than the disease.

This holistic approach extends to the mental and emotional aspects of health. Hahnemann observed that emotional states such as grief or shock could significantly impact physical health, a perspective that was innovative for his time. Homeopathy views disease as a disturbance of the body's vital force, with remedies aiming to stimulate this vital energy to restore balance and health.

The practice of homeopathy spread as Hahnemann's students and followers continued to practice and teach his methods. By the early 19th century, homeopathy had taken root in Europe and America, offering a gentler alternative to the often harsh and invasive medical practices of the time. Hahnemann's meticulous documentation and the publication of his works, such as "The Organon of the Healing Art," played a crucial role in disseminating his ideas. The "Organon" outlined the principles of homeopathy and provided practical guidelines for its practice, becoming the foundational text for homeopathic practitioners.

The Art of Dilution: Potentization and Succussion

In homeopathy, potentization and succession are pivotal processes transforming substances into therapeutic agents. Potentization involves systematic dilution, often to a point where no molecules of the starting material are detectable, combined with succession to transfer the substance's essence or 'energy' into the medium (water or alcohol). Hahnemann developed these methods to mitigate the toxic effects observed with undiluted substances, discovering that the curative properties persisted and were even enhanced through dilution and succussion.

This methodology challenges conventional pharmacology, which relies on dose-dependent effects. The theory behind potentization suggests that the process imprints the memory of the substance onto the diluent, interacting with the body's vital force. Each level of dilution, known as potency, is marked by a specific ratio, and the choice of potency is tailored to the individual patient based on their symptoms.

Succussion is believed to activate the medicinal properties of the solution. Despite skepticism from mainstream science regarding the mechanisms by which succussion enhances therapeutic efficacy, practitioners and patients attest to its qualitative difference, suggesting that shaking is integral to remedy preparation.

The concept of potentization extends beyond remedy preparation to reflect a broader holistic approach. It underscores that the remedy's effectiveness lies not only in its substance but also in its preparation and administration, emphasizing a process-oriented approach to healing. Hahnemann's theory of potentization was not static; he continued to refine and improve his methods throughout his life. His later works, such as the sixth edition of "The Organon," introduced the concept of using even higher dilutions (LM potencies), which he believed could achieve deeper and more lasting healing effects.

Potentization also embodies the homeopathic respect for the complexity and sensitivity of the body. It operates on the understanding that very subtle triggers can activate the body's healing mechanisms and that these mechanisms are capable of profound responses. The tailored potencies speak to this sensitivity, offering a spectrum of stimuli that can be matched to the individual's health and vitality.

The Principle of the Minimum Dose

The principle of the minimum dose in homeopathy posits that the lowest amount of a substance needed to initiate a healing response is the most desirable dosage. This principle aims to avoid side effects and supports the body's natural healing processes without overpowering or suppressing them. Hahnemann sought a gentle and respectful approach to healing, contrasting with the harsh methods of conventional treatments.

The minimum dose principle operates in tandem with potentization to produce remedies interacting with the body's vital force rather than directly affecting its physiology. The goal is to provide enough stimulus for the body's healing response without causing aggravation, reflecting a patient-centered approach that respects the body's pace and capacity for recovery.

Critics argue that minute doses, often beyond the presence of the original substance, cannot have any effect. However, homeopaths assert that clinical outcomes justify their approach, calling for an expanded understanding of drug action beyond material dose-response relationships.

The principle of the minimum dose also speaks to a philosophical stance recognizing the body as a self-healing organism, with medicine supporting rather than usurping the healing process. This principle remains a cornerstone of homeopathic medicine, emphasizing gentle intervention and respect for the body's inherent healing capabilities. The principle aligns with modern trends towards personalized medicine and the minimization of pharmacological interventions, reflecting a growing recognition of the need for more individualized and less invasive therapeutic approaches.

The Individualized Approach: The Patient as the Central Focus

The individualized approach in homeopathy views each patient as a unique entity requiring a tailored treatment strategy. Unlike the standardized protocols of conventional medicine, homeopathy emphasizes comprehensive assessment of the patient's physical, emotional, and mental symptoms, along with their medical history and life circumstances.

This approach demands thorough case-taking, with homeopaths conducting in-depth interviews to understand the patient's subtle symptoms and responses to various influences. The detailed questioning explores aspects such as food preferences, sleep patterns, and emotional temperament, which are crucial in selecting the most fitting remedy.

The individualized approach acknowledges the complexity of the human condition, respecting that the manifestations of illness are as diverse as the people experiencing them. Effective treatment must resonate with the patient's overall well-being, stimulating the body's healing processes in alignment with the individual's vitality and health.

Homeopaths view this approach to honor the whole person, addressing mental and emotional health as integral components of overall well-being. This dynamic process is responsive to changes in the patient's symptoms and health status, allowing for a flexible and evolving treatment strategy. This individualization extends to chronic conditions, where homeopaths may adjust remedies over time to reflect the shifting nature of the patient's health and circumstances.

Moreover, the individualized approach in homeopathy involves creating a therapeutic partnership between the practitioner and the patient. Homeopaths invest significant time in understanding the patient's life story, experiences, and personality traits, fostering a deeper connection that enhances the healing process. This relationship is built on trust, empathy, and mutual respect, providing a supportive environment for patients to engage actively in their healing journey.

The Holistic Philosophy: Treating the Whole Person

The holistic philosophy in homeopathy involves treating the individual in their entirety, considering the complex interplay between mind, body, and spirit. This approach views symptoms as expressions of the body's attempt to heal itself and emphasizes restoring balance within the whole person.

In practice, this philosophy involves meticulous consideration of the patient's physical symptoms, emotional state, mental health, and life circumstances. Homeopaths believe that emotional disturbances or life stressors can manifest as physical ailments, and vice versa, necessitating a comprehensive evaluation.

By addressing the person, homeopathy aims to bring about a state of harmony where health can flourish on all levels. Remedies are intended to support the body's self-healing mechanisms, encouraging a return to balance rather than merely suppressing symptoms.

The holistic approach extends to understanding and treating chronic illnesses, where symptoms can be complex and multifaceted. Homeopathy seeks to understand the underlying patterns of sustaining illness, working towards a sustainable and long-term restoration of health. This approach also involves preventative measures, promoting lifestyle changes that support overall well-being and reduce the likelihood of disease recurrence.

Homeopathy's holistic philosophy aligns with contemporary integrative medicine practices, which advocate for a comprehensive approach to health that includes diet, exercise, stress management, and mental health support. Homeopaths often provide guidance on these aspects, recognizing that a balanced lifestyle is crucial for maintaining health and preventing disease.

The Dynamis Concept: Vital Force as the Essence of Life

The concept of vital force, also known as vital energy, is fundamental to homeopathy's understanding of health and disease. It posits that a dynamic energy force animates all living beings, governing their physical functions and adaptive processes. When this vital force is imbalanced, it leads to symptoms of illness, and homeopathic remedies aim to stimulate this energy to restore balance.

This vitalist perspective differentiates homeopathy from conventional Western medicine, which is primarily mechanical and biochemical. Homeopaths assert that the vital force, although not directly observable, is discernible by its effects. The state of the vital force is reflected in the individual's overall well-being, including their mental, emotional, and physical conditions.

In practice, homeopaths seek to match the remedy's energy with the patient's disturbed vital force. This interaction is believed to stimulate the self-healing process. Symptoms are seen as expressions of a disturbed vital force, guiding the selection of an appropriate remedy to address the underlying imbalance.

The vital force concept is central to homeopathy's holistic treatment of patients, recognizing that symptoms indicate a more profound disturbance rather than merely organ dysfunction. It aligns with other traditional healing systems, such as qi in Traditional Chinese Medicine or prana in Ayurveda, emphasizing the balance of life energy for good health.

Various factors, including emotional states, environmental conditions, and lifestyle choices, influence the strength and harmony of the vital force. Therefore, a homeopath may guide diet, stress management, and other aspects of life that can support the patient's vitality. Maintaining a robust and balanced vital force is critical to resilience against illness.

In dealing with chronic diseases, the concept of the vital force is particularly significant. Homeopaths consider the long-term vitality and energy patterns of the individual, aiming to gradually restore the disturbed vital force to a state of equilibrium. Chronic symptoms indicate a deep-seated imbalance in the vital force that requires a sustained therapeutic strategy.

The vital force concept also informs the homeopathic perspective on prevention. A well-balanced vital energy confers immunity and resilience, reducing disease susceptibility. Thus, homeopathy places a strong emphasis on strengthening the vital force as a means of preventing illness and promoting long-term health.

The Principle of Potentization: Unlocking Remedial Energy

The principle of potentization is a hallmark of homeopathy, representing a unique process by which remedies are prepared to enhance their healing properties. This involves serial dilution and succussion (vigorous shaking) of a substance, aiming to release its energetic potential. Homeopaths believe this process amplifies the remedy's therapeutic qualities, stimulating the body's vital force while minimizing toxic side effects.

Potentization challenges conventional dose-response relationships, suggesting that the therapeutic qualities of a substance can operate at a level subtler than the molecular or chemical. The process is thought to imprint the substance's "memory" onto the diluent, with each dilution and succussion step increasing this energetic imprint.

The choice of potency is critical and tailored to each patient, considering factors such as sensitivity, illness nature, and symptom duration. The meticulous preparation of remedies reflects homeopathy's respect for both the material and non-material aspects of healing.

Potentization is not merely a means of remedy preparation but also a philosophical stance on the nature of medicine and healing. It posits that energy and information are central to health and that substances have capacities beyond their chemical composition. These principles challenge conventional medical paradigms and invite a broader understanding of what is therapeutically possible.

Homeopaths argue that potentization allows for a more precise and personalized approach to treatment. By selecting the appropriate potency, practitioners can tailor the remedy to the individual needs of the patient, ensuring that the treatment is both effective and gentle.

This personalized approach is a testament to the detailed nature of homeopathic practice and its commitment to individualized care.

The Doctrine of Drug Proving: Understanding Remedies through Human Experience

The Doctrine of Drug Proving is fundamental to homeopathy, whereby substances are systematically tested on healthy individuals to determine the range of symptoms they produce. These symptoms are meticulously cataloged to create detailed remedy profiles, ensuring therapeutic applications are grounded in empirical observation and direct human experience.

Drug proving involves healthy volunteers taking a homeopathic potency of a substance and recording all changes experienced. These self-observations contribute to the homeopathic materia medica, guiding the selection of remedies to match patient symptoms.

The methodology emphasizes safety, with remedies used in highly diluted forms to minimize adverse effects. Drug proving reflects homeopathy's empirical approach, respecting the nuances of human experiences and emphasizing the importance of subjective reports as valuable diagnostic tools.

The records from drug provings are compiled and scrutinized by homeopaths to discern patterns and characteristic symptoms that are consistently produced by the substance. These typical symptoms become essential in the homeopathic prescription process as they guide the practitioner in matching a patient's symptoms with the remedy profile.

The Doctrine of Drug Proving is also a testament to the homeopathic respect for the subtlety of human perception and the complexity of human experiences. Unlike conventional trials that may dismiss subjective experiences as irrelevant or anecdotal, homeopathy values these personal reports as essential data for understanding the multi-dimensional impact of remedies.

Drug proving is an ongoing process, reflecting homeopathy's openness to discovering new remedies and expanding its materia medica. As society encounters new substances and our environments change, homeopathy recognizes the need to explore and understand the healing potential of new agents continuously.

Summary of this chapter

Homeopathic medicine represents a unique and distinct paradigm within the broader field of medical sciences, characterized by its foundational principles, historical context, and philosophical underpinnings. This summary provides a comprehensive overview of the salient features of homeopathy, reflecting its evolution and enduring relevance in contemporary healthcare.

Homeopathy originated in the late 18th century through the pioneering work of Samuel Hahnemann, a German physician who sought alternatives to the harsh and often ineffective medical practices of his time. Dissatisfied with conventional treatments such as bloodletting and purging, Hahnemann formulated the principle of "similia similibus curentur" or "like cures like." This doctrine posits that substances capable of producing symptoms in healthy individuals can be utilized to treat similar symptoms in the sick, thus stimulating the body's intrinsic healing mechanisms. This foundational concept marked a significant departure from the prevailing medical theories and practices, setting the stage for the development of a new therapeutic system.

Central to homeopathy is the process of potentization, which involves the serial dilution and succussion (vigorous shaking) of substances to enhance their therapeutic properties while minimizing toxicity. This method, which imprints the "memory" of the original substance onto the diluent, challenges conventional pharmacological principles. However, it remains a cornerstone of homeopathic practice, reflecting a nuanced understanding of the interplay between substance, energy, and the body's vital force.

The principle of the minimum dose further distinguishes homeopathy from conventional medicine. By advocating for the smallest possible amount of a substance to elicit a healing response, homeopathy emphasizes a gentle, patient-centered approach that avoids overwhelming the body's natural processes. This minimalistic strategy aligns with a broader philosophical stance that respects the body's inherent wisdom and self-regulatory capabilities.

Homeopathy's individualized approach to treatment underscores its commitment to personalized care. Unlike standardized protocols in conventional medicine, homeopathy tailors its remedies to the unique constellation of physical, emotional, and mental symptoms presented by each patient. This holistic perspective integrates various dimensions of health, recognizing the interconnectedness of the mind, body, and spirit. Such an approach is particularly valuable in managing chronic and complex conditions, where a deeper understanding of the patient's overall well-being is paramount.

The concept of vital force, or vital energy, is integral to homeopathy's theoretical framework. This vitalist perspective posits that health is maintained by a dynamic equilibrium of intrinsic energy, which, when disrupted, manifests as disease. Homeopathic remedies aim to restore balance to this vital force, a notion that resonates with various traditional healing systems worldwide, such as qi in Traditional Chinese Medicine and prana in Ayurveda.

The empirical basis of homeopathy is further reinforced by the Doctrine of Drug Proving. This methodology involves systematically testing substances on healthy individuals to document the full spectrum of symptoms they produce. These detailed observations form the materia medica, guiding practitioners in selecting remedies that match the patient's symptom profile. This rigorous, experiential approach underscores the importance of subjective reports as valuable diagnostic tools and ensures that homeopathic treatments are grounded in direct human experience.

In conclusion, homeopathic medicine offers a distinctive and holistic approach to healthcare, emphasizing individualized treatment, minimal dosing, and the restoration of vital force. Its principles challenge conventional medical paradigms, advocating for a patient-centered, gentle, and integrative approach to healing. By understanding these foundational concepts and their historical evolution, one gains a deeper appreciation of homeopathy's role and potential within the broader landscape of medical practice. This comprehensive overview underscores the enduring relevance and adaptability of homeopathic principles in addressing contemporary health challenges, reflecting a commitment to a more personalized and holistic vision of health and well-being.

Chapter 2: Materia Medica

Green Strawberry Quartz: Comprehensive Guide on Spiritual and Physical Healing Properties

Overview

Green Strawberry Quartz, distinguished by its enchanting green hue interspersed with seed-like speckles, is a variant of quartz revered for fostering heart-centered awareness. It is highly esteemed for its ability to enhance relationships and personal connections, emanating a soothing energy that pacifies the mind during tumultuous times.

Spiritual and Psychic Benefits

Heart-Centered Awareness: Green Strawberry Quartz opens and aligns the heart chakra, cultivating a profound sense of love and empathy. It encourages heart-led living, promoting compassion and understanding in personal interactions.

Enhancing Relationships: This gemstone is particularly effective in fortifying relationships. It deepens emotional connections and fosters a nurturing approach towards loved ones, making it ideal for those seeking to strengthen their personal bonds.

Calming Energy: The tranquil properties of Green Strawberry Quartz help to soothe the mind and alleviate stress. It is especially beneficial during emotional upheaval, providing a stabilizing effect that promotes mental clarity and peace.

Emotional Healing: Green Strawberry Quartz supports emotional healing by facilitating the release of past traumas and encouraging forgiveness, both of oneself and others. This aids in overcoming emotional wounds and moving forward with a positive outlook.

Personal Growth: By promoting heart-centered living, this stone supports personal growth and the development of a more empathetic and understanding character.

Physical Healing Properties

Stress Reduction: The calming effect of Green Strawberry Quartz is beneficial not only for mental and emotional health but also for alleviating physical symptoms associated with stress, such as tension headaches and fatigue.

Immune System Support: This stone is believed to enhance the immune system, providing a general boost to physical health and well-being.

Heart Health: Associated with the heart chakra, Green Strawberry Quartz may have beneficial effects on heart health, helping to regulate heart functions and promote cardiovascular well-being.

Detoxification: It supports the body's detoxification processes, aiding in the removal of toxins and contributing to overall vitality and health.

Skin Health: Green Strawberry Quartz is also thought to improve skin condition, helping to soothe irritation and promote a healthy glow.

Potential Homeopathic Uses

Psychological Symptoms: Useful for addressing issues related to emotional disconnect, relationship difficulties, and stress-related mental challenges.

Physical Symptoms: Supports immune system function, contributes to heart health, and aids in stress relief and detoxification.

Behavioral Symptoms: Encourages more heartfelt interactions, fosters emotional understanding, and helps maintain calm in turbulent situations.

Green Strawberry Quartz's homeopathic profile would focus on its ability to enhance heart-centered awareness and emotional connections, making it suitable for addressing a range of emotional and physical conditions related to stress and relationships.

Conclusion

Green Strawberry Quartz is a unique and beneficial gemstone in holistic healing, appreciated not only for its captivating appearance but also for its extensive healing properties. Whether used to foster better relationships, support emotional healing, or enhance physical health, Green Strawberry Quartz serves as a powerful aid in achieving a balanced and harmonious life. As with all alternative practices, these should be considered complementary to conventional medical treatments, integral to a holistic approach to health.

Ocean Jasper: Comprehensive Guide on Spiritual and Physical Healing Properties

Overview

Ocean Jasper, known for its orbicular patterns and vibrant, multi-colored designs, is a stone of joy and renewal. It is cherished for its ability to lift spirits, release negative feelings, and soothe the emotional body. This gemstone promotes self-love and encourages compassion towards others, making it a valuable ally in personal growth and interpersonal relationships.

Spiritual and Psychic Benefits

Elevated Spirits and Joy: Ocean Jasper is highly effective in promoting joy and positivity. It helps to elevate spirits and foster a sense of contentment and happiness, making it ideal for those experiencing sadness or depression.

Release of Negativity: This stone excels in absorbing and dispelling negative emotions. It cleanses the emotional body of pessimism, stress, and anxiety, replacing these feelings with optimism and peace.

Soothing Emotional Body: Ocean Jasper has a calming effect on the emotions. It helps stabilize the mood and soothe emotional wounds, providing comfort during times of stress or emotional upheaval.

Self-Love and Compassion: This gemstone encourages a deep sense of self-love and acceptance, promoting healthy self-esteem. It also enhances empathy and compassion towards others, fostering better personal and professional relationships.

Renewal: Ocean Jasper is associated with the renewal of spirit and energy. It encourages letting go of old habits and embracing new patterns of behavior that are more aligned with one's highest good.

Physical Healing Properties

Digestive Health: Ocean Jasper is believed to aid in the digestion process, helping to soothe digestive disorders and enhance nutrient absorption.

Detoxification: It supports the body's natural detoxification processes, aiding in the removal of toxins and promoting a healthier physical state.

Immune System Support: Ocean Jasper is thought to boost the immune system, enhancing the body's ability to fight off infections and diseases.

Circulatory System: This stone may help improve circulation, which in turn can enhance overall energy levels and vitality.

Stress-Related Conditions: Due to its calming effects, Ocean Jasper can be beneficial in treating conditions exacerbated by stress, such as hypertension and insomnia.

Potential Homeopathic Uses

Psychological Symptoms: Addresses issues such as depression, anxiety, and emotional distress. It also helps in overcoming negativity and fostering positive thinking.

Physical Symptoms: Supports digestive health, aids in detoxification, boosts immune function, and helps improve circulation.

Behavioral Symptoms: Encourages self-love, enhances compassion, and promotes emotional stability and renewal.

Ocean Jasper's homeopathic profile would focus on its ability to bring joy, release negativity, and soothe the emotional body, making it suitable for a wide range of conditions related to emotional health and physical well-being.

Conclusion

Ocean Jasper is a vital gemstone in holistic healing, appreciated not only for its beautiful appearance but also for its profound emotional and physical healing properties. Whether used to foster joy, promote emotional healing, or support physical health, Ocean Jasper serves as a powerful aid in achieving a balanced and healthy life. As with all alternative practices, these should be considered as complementary to conventional medical treatments, integral to a holistic approach to health.

Orange Moonstone: Comprehensive Guide on Spiritual and Physical Healing Properties

Overview

Orange Moonstone, characterized by its warm, orange hues that glow softly under light, is valued for its ability to enhance emotional expression and soothe emotional instability. This gemstone promotes positive well-being and rejuvenation of the emotional body, making it a favored choice for those seeking emotional balance and vitality.

Spiritual and Psychic Benefits

Emotional Expression: Orange Moonstone facilitates greater emotional expression and openness. It helps individuals communicate their feelings more clearly and confidently, fostering better personal relationships.

Soothing Emotional Instability: This stone has a calming effect on the emotional body, helping to stabilize mood swings and reduce stress. It is particularly beneficial for those who experience emotional turbulence or heightened sensitivity.

Positive Well-being: By promoting a sense of warmth and emotional nourishment, Orange Moonstone enhances overall well-being. It encourages optimism and helps to transform negative energy into positive outcomes.

Rejuvenation of the Emotional Body: Orange Moonstone supports the healing and rejuvenation of the emotional body. It aids in overcoming emotional scars from past experiences and fosters a fresh, positive approach to life.

Support for New Beginnings: This gemstone is often used to mark new beginnings and important transitions. Its nurturing energy provides support during times of change and encourages perseverance through challenges.

Physical Healing Properties

Digestive Health: Orange Moonstone is believed to positively affect the digestive system, helping to soothe digestive issues and promote healthy metabolism.

Hormonal Balance: It may also help in balancing hormonal cycles, making it useful for addressing issues related to menstruation and menopause.

Stress Relief: The soothing properties of Orange Moonstone can alleviate physical symptoms associated with stress, such as tension headaches or sleep disturbances.

Detoxification: This stone supports the body's natural detoxification processes, aiding in the elimination of toxins and contributing to overall physical health.

Immune System Enhancement: Orange Moonstone is thought to boost the immune system, providing additional protection against common illnesses.

Potential Homeopathic Uses

Psychological Symptoms: Addresses emotional instability, difficulties in expressing emotions, and tendencies toward negativity.

Physical Symptoms: Supports digestive health, aids in hormonal balance, and assists in stress-related ailments.

Behavioral Symptoms: Enhances emotional resilience, promotes positive thinking, and supports transitions and new beginnings.

Orange Moonstone's homeopathic profile would focus on its ability to enhance emotional expression, soothe instability, and promote overall emotional and physical well-being, making it suitable for a wide range of conditions related to emotional health and vitality.

Conclusion

Orange Moonstone is a significant gemstone in holistic healing, appreciated not only for its vibrant appearance but also for its extensive emotional and physical healing properties. Whether used to enhance emotional expression, support physical health, or aid in navigating life transitions, Orange Moonstone serves as a potent tool in achieving a balanced and fulfilling life. As with all alternative practices, these should be considered as complementary to conventional medical treatments, integral to a holistic approach to health.

Pearl Opal: Comprehensive Guide on Spiritual and Physical Healing Properties

Overview

Pearl Opal, known for its luminous sheen and soft, opalescent colors that mimic the appearance of pearls, is a gemstone cherished for its properties of inspiration, luck, and purity. It enhances personal integrity and helps to focus one's attention, making it a valuable stone for those seeking clarity and moral fortitude.

Spiritual and Psychic Benefits

Inspiration: Pearl Opal is highly regarded for its ability to spark inspiration. It stimulates the imagination and creativity, making it an excellent choice for artists, writers, and anyone involved in creative endeavors.

Luck and Prosperity: This stone is believed to attract good fortune and prosperity. It is often used by those seeking to enhance their luck in personal and professional pursuits.

Purity: Pearl Opal promotes a sense of purity and cleansing. It helps to clear the mind and spirit of negativity, fostering a pristine and unblemished outlook on life.

Personal Integrity: By enhancing personal integrity, Pearl Opal supports individuals in adhering to their moral and ethical principles. It strengthens character and encourages honesty and forthrightness.

Focus and Clarity: This gemstone aids in focusing attention and sharpening mental clarity. It helps to concentrate thoughts and make clear, decisive decisions, especially under pressure.

Physical Healing Properties

Emotional Healing: Pearl Opal is known for its soothing emotional effects. It can help alleviate emotional stress, reduce anxiety, and promote an overall sense of calm and well-being.

Respiratory Health: This stone may have benefits for respiratory health, helping to clear the airways and promote better breathing.

Detoxification: Pearl Opal supports the body's natural detoxification processes, aiding in the elimination of toxins and promoting a healthier physical state.

Hormonal Balance: It is also thought to help balance hormonal levels, which can stabilize mood swings and alleviate symptoms associated with hormonal imbalances.

Skin Health: Due to its purifying properties, Pearl Opal can benefit skin health, helping to improve the appearance of the skin and aid in the healing of various skin conditions.

Potential Homeopathic Uses

Psychological Symptoms: Addresses issues such as lack of inspiration, difficulty in maintaining personal integrity, and challenges in mental focus.

Physical Symptoms: Supports emotional healing, aids in respiratory function, assists in detoxification, and helps balance hormonal levels.

Behavioral Symptoms: Enhances personal and professional prosperity, promotes ethical behavior, and improves decision-making abilities.

Pearl Opal's homeopathic profile would focus on its ability to inspire and purify, making it suitable for addressing a range of emotional, physical, and spiritual issues.

Conclusion

Pearl Opal is a distinguished gemstone in holistic healing, appreciated not only for its striking appearance but also for its profound inspiring and purifying properties. Whether used to stimulate creativity, enhance personal integrity, or support physical and emotional health, Pearl Opal serves as a powerful aid in achieving a balanced and enriched life. As with all alternative practices, these should be considered as complementary to conventional medical treatments, integral to a holistic approach to health.

Persian Agate: Comprehensive Guide on Spiritual and Physical Healing Properties

Overview

Persian Agate, recognized for its diverse color patterns and grounding properties, is a versatile stone that balances physical, emotional, and intellectual energies. It is particularly valued for its ability to aid in overcoming negativity and bitterness, promoting a sense of well-being and inner stability.

Spiritual and Psychic Benefits

Grounding: Persian Agate provides strong grounding energy, helping individuals to maintain a stable and balanced presence. It anchors the spirit, allowing for a deeper connection to the physical world and a sense of security.

Balancing Energies: This stone harmonizes the physical, emotional, and intellectual energies, facilitating a balanced state that enhances overall functioning and well-being.

Overcoming Negativity: Persian Agate is effective in dispelling negative emotions such as bitterness and resentment. It encourages the release of anger and fosters forgiveness, leading to emotional healing and personal growth.

Intellectual Clarity: By promoting intellectual balance, Persian Agate enhances analytical capabilities and decision-making skills. It supports clear thinking and problem-solving, making it useful for those facing challenging decisions.

Emotional Stability: This gemstone helps stabilize the emotions, preventing overreactions and promoting a calm, composed demeanor.

Physical Healing Properties

Digestive Health: Persian Agate is believed to aid in the health of the digestive system, helping to soothe stomach issues and enhance digestion.

Circulatory System: It may also support the circulatory system, improving blood flow and overall vascular health.

Skin Health: This stone is associated with skin health, helping to improve the appearance of the skin and aid in healing skin disorders.

Detoxification: Persian Agate supports the body's natural detoxification processes, aiding in the removal of toxins and promoting a healthier physical state.

Immune System Enhancement: It is thought to boost the immune system, providing additional protection against infections and illnesses.

Potential Homeopathic Uses

Psychological Symptoms: Addresses issues such as emotional imbalance, intellectual confusion, and negative emotions like bitterness and anger.

Physical Symptoms: Supports digestive and circulatory health, assists in skin healing, and aids in detoxification.

Behavioral Symptoms: Enhances analytical skills, improves decision-making, and promotes emotional and intellectual stability.

Persian Agate's homeopathic profile would focus on its grounding and balancing properties, making it suitable for addressing a range of conditions related

to emotional, intellectual, and physical health.

Conclusion

Persian Agate is a significant gemstone in holistic healing, appreciated not only for its aesthetic beauty but also for its extensive grounding and balancing properties. Whether used to enhance emotional stability, support physical health, or improve intellectual clarity, Persian Agate serves as a potent tool in achieving a balanced and healthy life. As with all alternative practices, these should be considered as complementary to conventional medical treatments, integral to a holistic approach to health.

Phantom Quartz: Comprehensive Guide on Spiritual and Physical Healing Properties

Overview

Phantom Quartz, known for its distinctive ghost-like inclusions that appear like phantoms within the crystal, is celebrated for its profound metaphysical properties. It is highly valued for its ability to reveal the layers and dimensions of one's life over time, making it an excellent tool for enhancing meditation, clarifying life goals, and assisting in spiritual evolution.

Spiritual and Psychic Benefits

Revealing Life's Layers: Phantom Quartz is unique in its ability to reveal historical layers and phases of one's life, allowing for reflection on past lessons and growth. This quality makes it an excellent stone for understanding one's personal and spiritual development.

Enhancement of Meditation: This crystal deepens meditation practices by helping to clear the mind and connect with higher spiritual realms. It encourages inner silence and enhances the quality of meditative states.

Clarification of Life Goals: Phantom Quartz aids in clarifying life goals by helping individuals connect with their deeper purposes and intentions. It supports the alignment of one's actions with their true desires and aspirations.

Spiritual Evolution: By promoting understanding of oneself and the universe, Phantom Quartz facilitates spiritual growth and evolution. It helps individuals to ascend to higher states of consciousness and embrace their spiritual journey.

Healing of Old Wounds: This gemstone assists in the healing of old emotional wounds, helping to resolve past traumas that may be hindering current progress.

Physical Healing Properties

Immune System Support: Phantom Quartz is believed to enhance the immune system, providing a boost in overall health and protection against illness.

Detoxification: It supports the body's natural detoxification processes, aiding in the removal of toxins and contributing to better physical health.

Energy and Vitality: Phantom Quartz is known to increase energy levels and promote vitality, helping individuals feel rejuvenated and lively.

Pain Relief: This stone may also offer pain relief, particularly for chronic conditions, by helping to dissipate the pain's energy and soothe the affected areas.

Stress Reduction: Due to its calming properties, Phantom Quartz can alleviate stress and reduce symptoms related to anxiety and tension.

Potential Homeopathic Uses

Psychological Symptoms: Useful for addressing issues of stagnation, lack of direction, and unresolved past traumas.

Physical Symptoms: Supports immune system function, aids in detoxification, and assists in energy enhancement and pain relief.

Behavioral Symptoms: Enhances focus, encourages spiritual and personal growth, and helps in setting and achieving meaningful life goals.

Phantom Quartz's homeopathic profile would focus on its ability to reveal the deeper aspects of one's life and support spiritual and physical healing, making it suitable for a wide range of conditions related to personal development and health.

Conclusion

Phantom Quartz is a powerful gemstone in holistic healing, appreciated not only for its captivating appearance but also for its extensive healing properties. Whether used to enhance spiritual practices, support physical health, or foster personal growth, Phantom Quartz serves as a potent tool in achieving a balanced and insightful life. As with all alternative practices, these should be considered as complementary to conventional medical treatments, integral to a holistic approach to health.

Purple Green Agate: Comprehensive Guide on Spiritual and Physical Healing Properties

Overview

Purple Green Agate combines the stability and calm of purple with the balance and harmony of green. It is renowned for fostering creativity and encouraging the resolution of conflicts.

Spiritual and Psychic Benefits

Stability and Calm: The purple hues within this agate provide a sense of stability and calm, helping to soothe emotional turbulence and promote a tranquil state of mind.

Balance and Harmony: The green elements within the stone enhance balance and harmony, supporting a balanced lifestyle and fostering inner peace.

Creativity: Purple Green Agate is known to stimulate creativity, making it an excellent stone for artists, writers, and anyone involved in creative endeavors.

Conflict Resolution: This gemstone encourages the resolution of conflicts, both internal and external, promoting understanding and reconciliation.

Physical Healing Properties

Emotional Healing: Purple Green Agate aids in emotional healing, helping to alleviate stress and anxiety.

Detoxification: It supports the body's natural detoxification processes, aiding in the removal of toxins.

Immune System Support: This stone is believed to boost the immune system, enhancing the body's ability to fight off infections and illnesses.

Pain Relief: Purple Green Agate may also provide relief from physical pain, particularly headaches and joint discomfort.

Potential Homeopathic Uses

Psychological Symptoms: Useful for addressing emotional instability, stress, and creative blocks.

Physical Symptoms: Supports detoxification, immune function, and pain relief.

Behavioral Symptoms: Enhances creativity, promotes conflict resolution, and fosters emotional stability.

Purple Green Agate's homeopathic profile would focus on its ability to provide stability, balance, and creativity, making it suitable for a wide range of emotional, physical, and creative conditions.

Conclusion

Purple Green Agate is a versatile gemstone in holistic healing, appreciated for its unique combination of stability, balance, and creativity. Whether used to enhance emotional stability, support physical health, or stimulate creativity, Purple Green Agate serves as a potent tool in achieving a balanced and fulfilling life. As with all alternative practices, these should be considered as complementary to conventional medical treatments, integral to a holistic approach to health.

Purple Green Agate - This stone combines the stability and calm of purple with the balance and harmony of green, fostering creativity and encouraging the resolution of conflicts.

Purple Green Agate: Comprehensive Guide on Spiritual and Physical Healing Properties

Overview

Purple Green Agate, a vibrant gemstone exhibiting hues of both purple and green, uniquely combines the qualities of stability, calm, balance, and harmony. This stone is celebrated for its ability to foster creativity and encourage the resolution of conflicts, making it an excellent choice for those seeking to enhance their artistic abilities and interpersonal relationships.

Spiritual and Psychic Benefits

Stability and Calm: The purple aspect of this agate brings a sense of stability and calm, helping to soothe the mind and reduce anxiety. It is particularly beneficial during times of stress or when confronting emotional disturbances.

Balance and Harmony: The green in the stone promotes balance and harmony, aligning the emotional, physical, and intellectual states. This can enhance personal well-being and promote more harmonious relationships.

Fostering Creativity: Purple Green Agate stimulates the imagination and creativity, making it a valuable tool for artists, writers, and anyone engaged in creative pursuits. It encourages innovative thinking and the expression of ideas.

Conflict Resolution: This gemstone aids in resolving conflicts by promoting understanding and encouraging communication. It helps individuals see different perspectives and find common ground.

Enhanced Decision-Making: By combining calm with balance, Purple Green Agate assists in clear decision-making. It enables one to weigh various options and make choices that reflect a balanced approach.

Physical Healing Properties

Emotional Healing: The soothing properties of this agate help in healing emotional wounds, providing comfort and reducing feelings of sadness or grief.

Digestive Health: Purple Green Agate is believed to aid in the health of the digestive system, helping to soothe stomach ailments and enhance digestion.

Immune System Support: This stone may boost the immune system, enhancing the body's ability to fight off infections and maintain good health.

Skin Health: The calming effects of Purple Green Agate can also benefit the skin, helping to improve its condition and soothe skin irritations.

Detoxification: It supports the body's natural detoxification processes, aiding in the removal of toxins and promoting a healthier physical state.

Potential Homeopathic Uses

Psychological Symptoms: Addresses issues such as emotional imbalance, creative blocks, and difficulties in conflict resolution.

Physical Symptoms: Supports digestive health, boosts immune function, aids in skin healing, and assists in detoxification.

Behavioral Symptoms: Enhances creativity, promotes effective communication, and facilitates problem-solving and decision-making.

Purple Green Agate's homeopathic profile would focus on its ability to bring stability, balance, and creativity, making it suitable for a range of conditions related to emotional health, physical well-being, and interpersonal interactions.

Conclusion

Purple Green Agate is a significant gemstone in holistic healing, appreciated not only for its striking appearance but also for its broad spectrum of healing properties. Whether used to enhance creativity, support physical health, or foster harmony in relationships, Purple

Green Agate serves as a potent tool in achieving a balanced and enriched life. As with all alternative practices, these should be considered as complementary to conventional medical treatments, integral to a holistic approach to health.

Red Aventurine: Comprehensive Guide on Spiritual and Physical Healing Properties

Overview

Red Aventurine, known for its rich red color and sparkling inclusions, is a dynamic gemstone that promotes vitality, mental alertness, and creativity. It enhances determination, empowering individuals to face life's challenges with confidence and drive.

Spiritual and Psychic Benefits

Vitality and Energy: Red Aventurine is highly valued for its ability to boost physical vitality and energy, making it ideal for those who may feel lethargic or unmotivated. It energizes the body and spirit, encouraging a zest for life.

Mental Alertness: This stone enhances cognitive functions, including concentration and perception, aiding in mental clarity and alertness. It is beneficial for those needing to stay mentally sharp and focused.

Creativity: Red Aventurine stimulates creative thinking and problem-solving abilities. It encourages innovative ideas and helps break through creative blocks, making it a favorite among artists, writers, and anyone engaged in creative projects.

Determination: The gemstone strengthens determination and perseverance. It supports individuals in pursuing their goals with steadfastness and resilience, particularly during challenging times.

Confidence: By boosting self-confidence, Red Aventurine enables one to approach various situations with assurance and courage, helping to overcome doubts and insecurities.

Physical Healing Properties

Circulatory Health: Red Aventurine is believed to enhance blood circulation, which can improve energy levels and promote overall physical health.

Muscle Recovery: This stone aids in muscle recovery and reduces physical fatigue, making it useful for athletes or those involved in physically demanding activities.

Immune System Support: Red Aventurine may boost the immune system, helping to protect against illness and speed up recovery from common health issues.

Enhanced Metabolism: It is also associated with improving metabolism, aiding in energy production and weight management.

Detoxification: Red Aventurine supports the body's natural detoxification processes, helping to cleanse the liver and kidneys and promoting overall bodily health.

Potential Homeopathic Uses

Psychological Symptoms: Addresses issues such as lack of energy, creative inhibition, and low self-confidence.

Physical Symptoms: Supports circulatory health, aids muscle recovery, enhances immune function, and assists in metabolic and detoxification processes.

Behavioral Symptoms: Encourages proactive behavior, bolsters determination to overcome challenges, and promotes creative problem-solving.

Red Aventurine's homeopathic profile would focus on its ability to energize both mind and body, enhance creativity, and foster a confident, determined attitude, making it suitable for a range of conditions related to energy levels, mental clarity, and personal empowerment.

Conclusion

Red Aventurine is a significant gemstone in holistic healing, appreciated not only for its striking appearance but also for its extensive healing properties. Whether used to enhance physical vitality, stimulate creativity, or boost confidence, Red Aventurine serves as a powerful aid in achieving a balanced and vibrant life. As with all alternative practices, these should be considered as complementary to conventional medical treatments, integral to a holistic approach to health.

Red Jasper: Comprehensive Guide on Spiritual and Physical Healing Properties

Overview

Red Jasper, with its deep, earthy red hues, is a robust and protective gemstone known for enhancing endurance, strength, and stamina. It is revered for its grounding properties and is particularly beneficial during challenging times, providing emotional endurance and resilience.

Spiritual and Psychic Benefits

Endurance and Strength: Red Jasper is celebrated for its ability to bolster physical strength and endurance. It is ideal for those who require extra stamina in their daily activities or during physically demanding tasks.

Emotional Stability: This stone enhances emotional endurance, helping individuals maintain a calm and stable demeanor during stressful situations. It is particularly useful for navigating difficult emotional landscapes.

Grounding: Red Jasper provides strong grounding energy, connecting the bearer to the Earth and promoting a sense of stability and balance in life.

Courage and Insight: It fosters courage and promotes insight into personal difficulties, encouraging an honest assessment of one's challenges and the ability to overcome them.

Energy Boost: Red Jasper stimulates the base chakra, increasing vitality and enthusiasm for life. It helps awaken a renewed sense of energy and motivation.

Physical Healing Properties

Circulatory Health: Red Jasper is known to improve circulation, enhancing blood flow and revitalizing the body's energy systems.

Digestive System Support: This gemstone aids in digestive processes and can help in the detoxification of the organs, particularly the liver.

Immune System Enhancement: Red Jasper is thought to strengthen the immune system, providing support against illnesses and infections.

Pain Relief: It is also used to alleviate pain, particularly within the lower back, hips, and legs.

Stress Reduction: The calming properties of Red Jasper help mitigate the physical symptoms of stress, reducing tension and promoting overall well-being.

Potential Homeopathic Uses

Psychological Symptoms: Addresses issues such as lack of emotional resilience, fear, and indecision.

Physical Symptoms: Supports circulatory health, aids in digestion, boosts the immune system, and helps manage pain.

Behavioral Symptoms: Enhances determination, encourages a proactive approach to challenges, and promotes a balanced energy throughout the day.

Red Jasper's homeopathic profile would focus on its ability to provide physical and emotional endurance, enhance vitality, and promote a balanced and grounded state of being, making it suitable for a wide range of conditions related to physical health, mental stamina, and emotional stability.

Conclusion

Red Jasper is a vital gemstone in holistic healing, appreciated not only for its striking appearance but also for its extensive healing properties. Whether used to enhance physical stamina, support emotional resilience, or promote overall health, Red Jasper serves as a powerful aid in achieving a balanced and vigorous life. As with all alternative practices, these should be considered as complementary to conventional medical treatments, integral to a holistic approach to health.

Red Obsidian: Comprehensive Guide on Spiritual and Physical Healing Properties

Overview

Red Obsidian, characterized by its deep, translucent red color, is a potent gemstone known for its strong connection to the base chakra. It enhances grounding and balancing of energies, making it highly effective for those dealing with fears related to survival and financial independence.

Spiritual and Psychic Benefits

Base Chakra Stimulation: Red Obsidian is particularly adept at stimulating the base chakra, enhancing one's sense of grounding and connection to the physical world. This stimulation helps to foster a feeling of security and stability.

Overcoming Survival Fears: This stone is invaluable for those who are overcoming fears associated with basic survival needs such as financial independence and physical safety. It instills strength and resilience.

Energy Balancing: Red Obsidian helps balance body energies, aligning them with the earth's natural vibration. This balance is essential for maintaining both physical and emotional health.

Emotional Release: It aids in releasing deep-seated emotions and traumas, particularly those related to past fears and insecurities. This release allows for greater emotional freedom and healing.

Courage and Protection: Red Obsidian is known for its protective qualities, shielding the wearer from negative influences and providing the courage to face life's challenges head-on.

Physical Healing Properties

Enhanced Vitality: By stimulating the base chakra, Red Obsidian enhances physical vitality and energy, providing the stamina needed to tackle daily tasks.

Digestive Health: This gemstone is believed to aid in digestion and can help in resolving issues related to the gastrointestinal tract.

Detoxification: Red Obsidian supports the body's natural detoxification processes, helping to cleanse the blood and remove toxins that may impede health.

Immune System Support: It is thought to bolster the immune system, enhancing the body's ability to fight off infections and diseases.

Stress Reduction: The grounding properties of Red Obsidian help alleviate physical stress and tension, particularly in the muscles and nerves.

Potential Homeopathic Uses

Psychological Symptoms: Addresses issues such as anxiety over financial security, fear of physical harm, and emotional imbalances related to survival instincts.

Physical Symptoms: Supports digestive health, aids in detoxification, boosts immune function, and alleviates stress.

Behavioral Symptoms: Enhances personal courage, encourages emotional release, and promotes a balanced and grounded demeanor.

Red Obsidian's homeopathic profile would focus on its ability to stimulate the base chakra and balance energies, making it suitable for addressing a range of conditions related to physical and emotional security.

Conclusion

Red Obsidian is a significant gemstone in holistic healing, appreciated not only for its aesthetic appeal but also for its profound grounding and protective properties. Whether used to enhance physical health, support emotional stability, or overcome fears related to survival and independence, Red Obsidian serves as a potent tool in achieving a balanced and empowered life. As with all alternative practices, these should be considered as complementary to conventional medical treatments, integral to a holistic approach to health.

Red Rabbit Hair Quartz: Comprehensive Guide on Spiritual and Physical Healing Properties

Overview

Red Rabbit Hair Quartz, characterized by its captivating inclusions that resemble fine red threads or hairs within the crystal, is a unique and energizing gemstone. It is known for bringing warmth and energy, stimulating love and passion, and clearing negative emotional patterns, making it an excellent choice for those seeking emotional revitalization and personal transformation.

Spiritual and Psychic Benefits

Warmth and Energy: This stone is celebrated for its ability to infuse warmth and vitality into its surroundings. It energizes the spirit, encouraging enthusiasm and zest for life.

Stimulation of Love and Passion: Red Rabbit Hair Quartz is particularly effective in stimulating feelings of love and passion. It enhances romantic relationships and can help rekindle lost flames or deepen existing connections.

Clearing Negative Emotional Patterns: The gemstone has a powerful cleansing effect on emotional baggage, helping to dissolve old hurts and negative patterns that can hinder personal growth and happiness.

Emotional Healing: It supports deep emotional healing by promoting the release of repressed emotions and facilitating a healthier emotional expression.

Enhancing Creativity: The invigorating energy of Red Rabbit Hair Quartz also boosts creativity, making it useful for artists, writers, and anyone involved in creative endeavors.

Physical Healing Properties

Cardiovascular Health: Red Rabbit Hair Quartz is believed to benefit the heart by improving circulation and overall cardiovascular health.

Energy Boost: This quartz type enhances physical energy, making it beneficial for those dealing with fatigue or lethargy.

Stress Reduction: Its warming energy helps reduce stress and anxiety, promoting a sense of calm and well-being.

Detoxification: The stone supports the body's natural detoxification processes, aiding in the elimination of toxins and promoting a cleaner, healthier state.

Immune System Support: Red Rabbit Hair Quartz is thought to bolster the immune system, enhancing the body's ability to fight off illnesses and maintain good health.

Potential Homeopathic Uses

Psychological Symptoms: Addresses issues such as lack of passion, emotional coldness, and negative emotional cycles.

Physical Symptoms: Supports cardiovascular health, boosts energy levels, aids in detoxification, and enhances immune function.

Behavioral Symptoms: Promotes emotional openness, stimulates creativity, and fosters a more vibrant and passionate approach to life.

Red Rabbit Hair Quartz's homeopathic profile would focus on its ability to bring warmth and energy, stimulate emotional and physical well-being, and enhance creativity and passion, making it suitable for a range of conditions related to emotional health and physical vitality.

Conclusion

Red Rabbit Hair Quartz is a dynamic gemstone in holistic healing, appreciated not only for its striking visual appearance but also for its extensive healing properties. Whether used to stimulate love and passion, support physical health, or foster emotional and creative rejuvenation, Red Rabbit Hair Quartz serves as a powerful aid in achieving a balanced and fulfilling life. As with all alternative practices, these should be considered as complementary to conventional medical treatments, integral to a holistic approach to health.

Rutile Quartz: Comprehensive Guide on Spiritual and Physical Healing Properties

Overview

Rutile Quartz, distinguished by its needle-like rutile inclusions within a transparent quartz crystal, is a powerful stone known for its ability to attract love and stabilize relationships. It also aids in decision-making by helping its wearer overcome fear and doubt, making it a valuable ally in both personal and professional realms.

Spiritual and Psychic Benefits

Attracting Love: Rutile Quartz is particularly effective in drawing love into one's life. It opens the heart to both giving and receiving love and helps attract romantic partnerships that are supportive and fulfilling.

Stabilizing Relationships: This gemstone is excellent for stabilizing relationships and enhancing harmony between partners. It encourages honesty, understanding, and commitment, making it ideal for couples looking to deepen their connection.

Enhancing Decision-Making: Rutile Quartz supports clear and confident decision-making. It helps dispel fear and doubt, allowing for choices that are guided by wisdom and intuition rather than by anxiety or indecision.

Spiritual Growth: The stone aids in spiritual growth by amplifying spiritual insights and elevating one's consciousness. It facilitates a deeper connection with the divine and enhances meditative experiences.

Emotional Healing: Rutile Quartz helps in healing emotional wounds by promoting forgiveness and compassion. It supports emotional release and transformation, leading to greater inner peace.

Physical Healing Properties

Energy Boost: Rutile Quartz is known for its ability to increase energy and vitality. It helps combat fatigue and lethargy, providing a steady source of energy throughout the day.

Respiratory Health: This gemstone is believed to benefit the respiratory system, aiding in the treatment of bronchitis, asthma, and other respiratory conditions.

Immune System Support: Rutile Quartz may enhance the immune system, helping to protect against illness and speed up recovery from sickness.

Pain Relief: It is also known for its pain-relieving properties, particularly in cases of chronic conditions or injuries.

Detoxification: The stone supports the body's natural detoxification processes, aiding in the removal of toxins and promoting overall physical health.

Potential Homeopathic Uses

Psychological Symptoms: Addresses issues related to fear of commitment, difficulty in making decisions, and emotional traumas affecting relationships.

Physical Symptoms: Supports respiratory health, boosts energy levels, enhances immune function, and aids in pain management and detoxification.

Behavioral Symptoms: Promotes openness to love, stabilizes relationship dynamics, and encourages confident, fear-free decision-making.

Rutile Quartz's homeopathic profile would focus on its ability to attract and stabilize love, enhance decision-making, and support physical and emotional healing, making it suitable for a range of conditions related to personal growth and health.

Conclusion

Rutile Quartz is a significant gemstone in holistic healing, appreciated not only for its aesthetic beauty but also for its extensive healing properties. Whether used to enhance personal relationships, support physical health, or foster emotional and spiritual development, Rutile Quartz serves as a potent tool in achieving a balanced and enriched life. As with all alternative practices, these should be considered as complementary to conventional medical treatments, integral to a holistic approach to health.

Snowflake Obsidian: Comprehensive Guide on Spiritual and Physical Healing Properties

Overview

Snowflake Obsidian, distinguished by its dark, glassy luster punctuated with splotches of white resembling snowflakes, is a gemstone known for its calming and soothing properties. It helps put individuals in the right frame of mind to be receptive to new ideas and is celebrated for its purity and balancing effects on the body, mind, and spirit.

Spiritual and Psychic Benefits

Calming and Soothing: Snowflake Obsidian is highly effective in calming and soothing the mind, making it easier to handle stress and maintain a peaceful state of being. This tranquility is essential for mental clarity and receptiveness to new ideas.

Frame of Mind for Receptivity: This stone enhances the ability to be open and receptive to new ideas and experiences. It encourages flexibility in thinking and openness to new ways of problem-solving.

Purity: Known as a stone of purity, Snowflake Obsidian helps in the purification of the energy system, clearing it of negativity and psychic smog that can hinder personal growth and clarity.

Balance: It promotes balance among the physical, emotional, and spiritual aspects of life, helping to stabilize the mood and align inner energies with external demands.

Transformation: Snowflake Obsidian is also useful for promoting personal transformation, aiding in the recognition and release of outdated patterns and behaviors that no longer serve the individual.

Physical Healing Properties

Detoxification: This gemstone supports the body's natural detoxification processes, aiding in the elimination of toxins and promoting a healthier physical state.

Pain Relief: Snowflake Obsidian is known to help alleviate pain, especially muscular aches and spasms, contributing to overall comfort and physical wellbeing.

Circulatory Health: It may help improve circulation, enhancing blood flow and energy levels throughout the body.

Joint Health: The stone can also be beneficial for joint health, helping to reduce joint pain and discomfort.

Stress-Related Conditions: Due to its calming effects, Snowflake Obsidian can alleviate symptoms related to stress, such as hypertension and insomnia.

Potential Homeopathic Uses

Psychological Symptoms: Addresses issues such as stress, inability to focus, negative thought patterns, and emotional instability.

Physical Symptoms: Supports detoxification, provides pain relief, aids in improving circulation, and assists with joint health.

Behavioral Symptoms: Encourages openness to new ideas, promotes balance and harmony, and aids in the process of transformation and personal growth.

Snowflake Obsidian's homeopathic profile would focus on its ability to calm and soothe, promote receptivity and balance, and support physical healing, making it suitable for a wide range of conditions related to emotional and physical health.

Conclusion

Snowflake Obsidian is a valuable gemstone in holistic healing, appreciated not only for its distinctive appearance but also for its profound soothing and balancing properties. Whether used to enhance mental clarity, support physical health, or foster emotional and spiritual balance, Snowflake Obsidian serves as a powerful tool in achieving a balanced and harmonious life. As with all alternative practices, these should be considered as complementary to conventional medical treatments, integral to a holistic approach to health.

Southern Red Agate: Comprehensive Guide on Spiritual and Physical Healing Properties

Overview

Southern Red Agate, noted for its vibrant red tones and smooth, polished appearance, is a gemstone that enhances mental functions such as concentration, perception, and analytical abilities. It is also valued for its ability to help overcome personal challenges and enhance courage, making it a powerful tool for personal development and resilience.

Spiritual and Psychic Benefits

Enhanced Mental Functions: Southern Red Agate is particularly effective in boosting mental clarity and sharpness. It enhances concentration, aids in perception, and sharpens analytical abilities, which are crucial for problem-solving and decision-making.

Overcoming Challenges: This stone provides strength and support to overcome personal challenges and adversity. It instills resilience and perseverance, helping individuals to push through difficult circumstances and emerge stronger.

Boosting Courage: Southern Red Agate fosters courage and confidence, encouraging individuals to take bold steps and face their fears. It supports taking risks and stepping out of comfort zones, which is essential for personal growth.

Emotional Balance: Southern Red Agate helps stabilize the emotions, providing a soothing influence that can temper feelings of anger or distress. It promotes emotional wellness and stability.

Motivation: This gemstone is known for its ability to inspire and motivate, rekindling a passion for life's pursuits and encouraging a drive towards achieving personal goals.

Physical Healing Properties

Digestive Health: Southern Red Agate is believed to aid in the health of the digestive system, helping to soothe stomach ailments and enhance digestion.

Circulatory System: It may also support the circulatory system, improving blood flow and overall vascular health.

Enhanced Vitality: This stone boosts physical energy and vitality, helping to alleviate feelings of lethargy and fatigue.

Immune System Support: Southern Red Agate is thought to bolster the immune system, enhancing the body's ability to fend off illness and maintain good health.

Pain Relief: It can provide relief from physical pain, especially in the abdomen and lower back, contributing to overall comfort and well-being.

Potential Homeopathic Uses

Psychological Symptoms: Addresses issues such as lack of focus, poor analytical thinking, fearfulness, and low motivation.

Physical Symptoms: Supports digestive and circulatory health, enhances energy levels, boosts immune function, and aids in pain management.

Behavioral Symptoms: Encourages confidence, facilitates overcoming personal challenges, and promotes emotional stability and resilience.

Southern Red Agate's homeopathic profile would focus on its ability to enhance mental functions, support physical health, and foster personal development, making it suitable for a range of conditions related to mental clarity, emotional balance, and overall well-being.

Conclusion

Southern Red Agate is a significant gemstone in holistic healing, appreciated not only for its striking appearance but also for its extensive supportive properties. Whether used to enhance mental acuity, support physical health, or foster emotional and personal resilience, Southern Red Agate serves as a potent tool in achieving a balanced and fulfilling life. As with all alternative practices, these should be considered as complementary to conventional medical treatments, integral to a holistic approach to health.

Strawberry Quartz: Comprehensive Guide on Spiritual and Physical Healing Properties

Overview

Strawberry Quartz, known for its pink hues interspersed with specks and swirls that resemble strawberries, is a gemstone celebrated for stimulating the heart center and infusing one's entire being with the feeling of love. It promotes an aura of love and brings the euphoria of a truly loving environment, making it a powerful stone for emotional healing and personal growth.

Spiritual and Psychic Benefits

Heart Center Stimulation: Strawberry Quartz is particularly effective at stimulating the heart chakra, enhancing one's ability to give and receive love. It opens the heart to love from others and encourages self-love and acceptance.

Feeling of Love and Euphoria: This gemstone fosters an intense feeling of love and joy within one's environment. It helps create and enhance connections with others through empathy and understanding, contributing to a loving and supportive atmosphere.

Emotional Healing: Strawberry Quartz aids in the healing of emotional wounds by encouraging a positive outlook and replacing negative emotions with love and serenity. It can help soothe a troubled heart and bring relief from emotional distress.

Enhanced Intuition: By activating the heart chakra, Strawberry Quartz also enhances intuition, particularly in understanding interpersonal relationships and emotional dynamics. This heightened sensitivity can lead to better decision-making in personal interactions.

Promotion of Harmony: This stone promotes harmony and peace, both internally and in one's external relationships. It helps resolve conflicts and encourages compassionate and understanding communication.

Physical Healing Properties

Stress Reduction: The soothing energy of Strawberry Quartz can significantly reduce stress levels, helping to alleviate anxiety and tension.

Circulatory Health: This gemstone is believed to benefit the circulatory system, enhancing blood flow and contributing to overall heart health.

Skin Health: Strawberry Quartz can also improve the condition of the skin, promoting a healthy glow and aiding in the healing of skin issues related to emotional stress.

Immune System Support: It may enhance the immune system, providing a boost in overall health and resilience against illness.

Detoxification: Strawberry Quartz supports the body's natural detoxification processes, aiding in the elimination of toxins and promoting a healthier physical state.

Potential Homeopathic Uses

Psychological Symptoms: Addresses issues such as lack of affection, emotional coldness, and difficulties in personal relationships.

Physical Symptoms: Supports circulatory health, aids in stress relief, assists with skin health, and boosts immune function.

Behavioral Symptoms: Encourages open and loving communication, promotes emotional understanding, and fosters a sense of peace and harmony in interactions.

Strawberry Quartz's homeopathic profile would focus on its ability to stimulate feelings of love and emotional well-being, making it suitable for a range of conditions related to emotional health and physical balance.

Conclusion

Strawberry Quartz is a valuable gemstone in holistic healing, appreciated not only for its beautiful appearance but also for its profound emotional and physical healing properties. Whether used to enhance feelings of love, support physical health, or foster emotional and relational harmony, Strawberry Quartz serves as a powerful aid in achieving a balanced and loving life. As with all alternative practices, these should be considered as complementary to conventional medical treatments, integral to a holistic approach to health.

Tiger Iron: Comprehensive Guide on Spiritual and Physical Healing Properties

Overview

Tiger Iron, an intriguing amalgamation of Jasper, Hematite, and Tiger's Eye, is acclaimed for its ability to invigorate vitality and assist individuals in surmounting arduous phases of life. This gemstone is equally esteemed for its physical health benefits, including the equilibrium of red and white blood cell counts, the fortification of muscles, and the enhancement of stamina.

Spiritual and Psychic Benefits

Vitality and Energy: Tiger Iron is a stone imbued with strength and vitality, delivering an energy boost that can rejuvenate and invigorate. It is particularly advantageous for those experiencing physical or mental exhaustion.

Navigating Life Challenges: This gemstone offers robust support during challenging times, fostering resilience and perseverance. It aids individuals in remaining grounded and focused, even amidst tumultuous periods.

Emotional Stability: Tiger Iron stabilizes emotions, mitigating fears and anxiety. It fosters a balanced emotional state, essential for confronting life's challenges with confidence.

Enhanced Willpower: This stone amplifies determination and willpower, assisting individuals in overcoming obstacles and achieving their aspirations. It inspires a resilient spirit and a positive outlook.

Grounding: Integrating the grounding attributes of Jasper and Hematite with the protective qualities of Tiger's Eye, Tiger Iron is exemplary for grounding and safeguarding against negative influences.

Physical Healing Properties

Blood Health: Tiger Iron is reputed for balancing red and white blood cell counts, thereby supporting overall blood health and the body's intrinsic healing processes.

Muscle Strengthening: This gemstone bolsters muscle strength and enhances physical power and endurance, making it suitable for athletes or individuals engaged in physically demanding activities.

Improved Stamina: Tiger Iron augments stamina, facilitating sustained physical activity and maintaining energy levels throughout.

Pain Relief: The Hematite component of Tiger Iron is known to alleviate pain, particularly muscle strain or injuries.

Enhanced Respiratory Capacity: This stone may also improve respiratory health, aiding in better oxygen intake and supporting lung function.

Potential Homeopathic Uses

Psychological Symptoms: Addresses issues such as energy depletion, difficulty coping with stress, and emotional instability.

Physical Symptoms: Supports blood health, muscle strength, stamina, pain relief, and respiratory function.

Behavioral Symptoms: Encourages perseverance through challenges, enhances focus and determination, and helps maintain a balanced emotional state during stressful periods.

Tiger Iron's homeopathic profile emphasizes its ability to enhance vitality, support physical health, and provide stability during life's challenges, making it suitable for a range of conditions related to both physical stamina and emotional resilience.

Conclusion

Tiger Iron is a significant gemstone in holistic healing, valued not only for its striking appearance but also for its extensive healing properties. Whether used to enhance physical vitality, support emotional stability, or foster resilience in facing life's difficulties, Tiger Iron serves as a potent tool in achieving a balanced and vigorous life. As with all alternative practices, these should be considered complementary to conventional medical treatments, integral to a holistic approach to health.

Tsavorite Garnet: Comprehensive Guide on Spiritual and Physical Healing Properties

Overview

Tsavorite Garnet, renowned for its vivid green hue, is a precious gemstone celebrated for its qualities of prosperity, abundance, and emotional healing. It stimulates the heart chakra, enhancing compassion, emotional well-being, and physical healing capacity. Tsavorite Garnet is ideal for those wishing to cultivate gratitude and a spirit of generosity.

Spiritual and Psychic Benefits

Prosperity and Abundance: Tsavorite Garnet is often associated with attracting prosperity and enhancing abundance in one's life. It encourages positivity and the flow of universal riches, making it popular for those seeking financial improvement or abundance in various life aspects.

Gratitude and Service: This gemstone fosters deep gratitude and a desire to serve others, promoting a generous spirit and the joy of sharing one's blessings with the world.

Heart Chakra Stimulation: Tsavorite Garnet strongly connects to the heart chakra, stimulating it to open up feelings of compassion and love towards oneself and others. It helps clear blockages in the heart chakra, allowing for a freer exchange of love and emotional warmth.

Enhanced Compassion: The stone's energy enhances empathy and understanding, fostering deeper relationships and kinder interactions with others.

Emotional Healing: Tsavorite Garnet is particularly effective in healing emotional wounds, providing comfort during times of distress and fostering resilience in overcoming sadness or grief.

Physical Healing Properties

Cardiovascular Health: By stimulating the heart chakra, Tsavorite Garnet is believed to benefit the heart and circulatory system, improving overall cardiovascular health.

Detoxification: This gemstone supports the body's natural detoxification processes, aiding in the removal of toxins and contributing to a healthier physical state.

Immune System Support: Tsavorite Garnet is thought to boost the immune system, enhancing the body's natural defenses against illness.

Stress Reduction: The calming properties of this stone help reduce stress and anxiety, promoting a sense of well-being and relaxation.

Energy and Vitality: Tsavorite Garnet enhances energy and vitality, providing a boost to physical health and stamina.

Potential Homeopathic Uses

Psychological Symptoms: Addresses issues such as lack of generosity, difficulties in experiencing joy, and emotional coldness.

Physical Symptoms: Supports cardiovascular health, aids in detoxification, boosts the immune system, reduces stress, and enhances overall vitality.

Behavioral Symptoms: Encourages acts of kindness, fosters emotional connections, and promotes an attitude of gratitude and service.

Tsavorite Garnet's homeopathic profile emphasizes its ability to stimulate prosperity, enhance emotional and physical health, and promote compassionate behaviors, making it suitable for a range of conditions related to emotional balance, physical health, and spiritual growth.

Conclusion

Tsavorite Garnet is a valuable gemstone in holistic healing, appreciated not only for its beauty but also for its extensive healing properties. Whether used to enhance financial prosperity, support physical and emotional health, or foster a spirit of generosity and compassion, Tsavorite Garnet serves as a powerful tool in achieving a balanced and enriched life. As with all alternative practices, these should be considered complementary to conventional medical treatments, integral to a holistic approach to health.

Vesuvianite: Comprehensive Guide on Spiritual and Physical Healing Properties

Overview

Vesuvianite, also known as Idocrase, is a gemstone celebrated for its ability to promote loyalty to humankind and stimulate creativity. It encourages the expression of one's true self, making it a powerful tool for personal authenticity and creative exploration. This stone is known for its vibrant green and brown hues, often found in proximity to volcanic regions.

Spiritual and Psychic Benefits

Promotion of Loyalty: Vesuvianite enhances feelings of loyalty, not only to individuals but to humanity as a whole. It fosters a sense of connection and commitment to the well-being of others, enhancing social cohesion and empathy.

Stimulation of Creativity: This gemstone effectively stimulates creativity, unlocking the creative process and aiding those in artistic fields to find new inspiration and express their ideas more freely.

Expression of True Self: Vesuvianite encourages the wearer to embrace and express their true self. It helps dismantle barriers preventing authenticity, enabling individuals to show their true colors and align their external life with their internal values.

Emotional Healing: The stone aids in releasing negative emotions and overcoming fears that inhibit self-expression. It promotes emotional clarity and stability, paving the way for a healthier emotional life.

Enhanced Decision-Making: By fostering alignment with one's true self, Vesuvianite aids in making decisions more in tune with one's deepest desires and needs, leading to greater personal satisfaction.

Physical Healing Properties

Support for Physical Vitality: Vesuvianite enhances physical vitality, invigorating the body and boosting overall energy levels.

Detoxification: This stone supports the body's detoxification processes, aiding in eliminating toxins and promoting a healthier physical state.

Strengthening of Teeth and Bones: Vesuvianite benefits the health of bones and teeth, potentially aiding in strengthening these structures and improving overall skeletal health.

Enhancement of Nutrient Absorption: It may also assist in better nutrient absorption, contributing to improved health and well-being.

Stress Reduction: Due to its calming properties, Vesuvianite helps reduce physical symptoms of stress, promoting relaxation and ease.

Potential Homeopathic Uses

Psychological Symptoms: Addresses issues such as disloyalty, lack of creativity, fear of self-expression, and emotional suppression.

Physical Symptoms: Supports general vitality, aids in detoxification, strengthens bones and teeth, and assists with nutrient absorption.

Behavioral Symptoms: Encourages authenticity, boosts creativity, and enhances commitment to communal and personal relationships.

Vesuvianite's homeopathic profile emphasizes its ability to promote loyalty, stimulate creativity, and encourage true self-expression, making it suitable for a range of conditions related to personal growth and physical health.

Conclusion

Vesuvianite is a significant gemstone in holistic healing, valued not only for its aesthetic appeal but also for its extensive healing properties. Whether used to enhance emotional and physical health, stimulate creativity, or foster authenticity and loyalty, Vesuvianite serves as a powerful tool in achieving a balanced and fulfilling life. As with all alternative practices, these should be considered complementary to conventional medical treatments, integral to a holistic approach to health.

Vivianite: Comprehensive Guide on Spiritual and Physical Healing Properties

Overview

Vivianite, with its deep blue to green hues, is a relatively rare gemstone known for its profound empathetic qualities. It fosters compassion and deep understanding, enabling individuals to genuinely perceive and relate to the emotions of others. This stone is particularly beneficial for aiding those undergoing emotional turmoil, providing support and clarity in navigating complex feelings.

Spiritual and Psychic Benefits

Enhancement of Compassion: Vivianite is highly effective in opening the heart chakra, enhancing one's capacity for compassion and empathy. It allows individuals to connect deeply with others' feelings and experiences, fostering understanding and supportive relationships.

Aid in Emotional Turmoil: This gemstone provides calm and clarity in times of emotional distress. It helps soothe the soul, offering relief from heavy emotional burdens and facilitating a path to emotional recovery.

Deep Emotional Insight: Vivianite encourages introspection and self-awareness, helping individuals understand the root causes of their emotions. This insight can lead to profound emotional healing and personal growth.

Strengthening Emotional Bonds: By promoting empathy and understanding, Vivianite strengthens emotional connections between people, making it ideal for healing strained relationships or enhancing close bonds.

Spiritual Growth: The stone aids in spiritual development by encouraging a compassionate and understanding approach to life's challenges, aligning one's actions with higher spiritual values.

Physical Healing Properties

Stress Reduction: Vivianite helps reduce stress and anxiety by calming the mind and soothing the nervous system. Its tranquil energy promotes a state of peace and relaxation.

Enhancement of Physical Vitality: Although subtle, Vivianite can contribute to increased physical energy and vitality, especially when emotional exhaustion depletes the body's resources.

Support for the Circulatory System: This stone is believed to aid in the health of the circulatory system, improving blood flow and overall cardiovascular health.

Detoxification: Vivianite supports the body's detoxification processes, aiding in the removal of toxins and promoting a healthier physical state.

Immune System Boost: The calming properties of Vivianite may indirectly support the immune system by reducing stress, which is known to impact immune health negatively.

Potential Homeopathic Uses

Psychological Symptoms: Addresses issues such as lack of empathy, emotional disconnect, and intense emotional turmoil.

Physical Symptoms: Supports stress relief, enhances vitality, aids circulatory health, assists in detoxification, and boosts immune function.

Behavioral Symptoms: Encourages more profound compassion in interpersonal interactions, aids in emotional understanding, and supports emotional resilience.

Vivianite's homeopathic profile emphasizes its ability to foster deep compassion, enhance emotional understanding, and support both emotional and physical healing, making it suitable for a range of conditions related to emotional health and interpersonal relationships.

Conclusion

Vivianite is a significant gemstone in holistic healing, appreciated not only for its unique beauty but also for its extensive emotional and physical healing properties. Whether used to enhance empathetic understanding, support emotional or physical health, or foster personal and spiritual growth, Vivianite serves as a powerful tool in achieving a balanced and compassionate life. As with all alternative practices, these should be considered complementary to conventional medical treatments, integral to a holistic approach to health.

White Coral: Comprehensive Guide on Spiritual and Physical Healing Properties

Overview

White Coral, distinguished by its delicate, pale coloration, is not a gemstone but an organic material formed by marine animals. It is revered for its ability to support diplomacy and conciliation, nurturing cooperation among individuals and expelling negativity. White Coral is often used in practices that require harmony and balance, making it an excellent choice for fostering peaceful interactions and environments.

Spiritual and Psychic Benefits

Diplomacy and Conciliation: White Coral enhances diplomatic skills, helping individuals communicate more effectively and conciliate disputes. It promotes understanding and respect among differing parties, making it ideal for resolving conflicts.

Nurturing Cooperation: This coral encourages a spirit of cooperation, making it useful in teamwork and group settings where harmonious interaction is crucial.

Expelling Negativity: White Coral has the ability to dispel negativity from both the environment and the mind. It promotes a positive atmosphere and helps maintain a clear, optimistic outlook.

Emotional Balance: It aids in achieving emotional balance, soothing feelings of tension and stress and replacing them with calmness and serenity.

Enhancing Intuition: White Coral can also help in enhancing intuitive abilities, particularly in understanding and resolving emotional conflicts.

Physical Healing Properties

Bone Strength: White Coral is traditionally believed to support bone health due to its calcium content. It may help in strengthening bones and supporting the body's skeletal structure.

Immune System Support: This coral is thought to enhance the immune system, providing a boost in overall health and protection against infections.

Stress Reduction: The calming properties of White Coral help reduce physical symptoms associated with stress, promoting relaxation and a sense of well-being.

Detoxification: White Coral supports the body's natural detoxification processes, aiding in the removal of toxins and promoting a healthier physical state.

Circulatory Health: It may also benefit the circulatory system, improving blood flow and contributing to cardiovascular health.

Potential Homeopathic Uses

Psychological Symptoms: Addresses issues such as difficulty in communication, inability to cooperate, and pervasive negativity.

Physical Symptoms: Supports bone health, boosts immune function, assists in stress relief, aids in detoxification, and enhances circulatory health.

Behavioral Symptoms: Encourages diplomacy, fosters cooperation in group settings, and promotes a positive and harmonious environment.

White Coral's homeopathic profile emphasizes its ability to support interpersonal relationships, promote emotional and physical health, and foster an environment free from negativity, making it suitable for a range of conditions related to personal interaction and overall well-being.

Conclusion

White Coral is a significant organic material in holistic healing, appreciated not only for its aesthetic appeal but also for its extensive supportive properties. Whether used to enhance interpersonal skills, support physical health, or promote emotional balance, White Coral serves as a powerful aid in achieving a balanced and harmonious life. As with all alternative practices, these should be considered complementary to conventional medical treatments, integral to a holistic approach to health.

Yellow Aventurine: Comprehensive Guide on Spiritual and Physical Healing Properties

Overview

Yellow Aventurine, often characterized by its translucent yellow hue, is a variant of Aventurine, a stone rich in quartz. It is celebrated for its ability to inspire understanding and creativity, and for promoting a positive, easy-going attitude towards life. This gemstone is valued for enhancing personal power and optimism, making it an excellent choice for those looking to foster both personal growth and a joyous disposition.

Spiritual and Psychic Benefits

Inspiration and Creativity: Yellow Aventurine stimulates the solar plexus chakra, which is associated with personal power and creativity. It encourages creative thinking and problem-solving, making it a great stone for artists, writers, and anyone involved in creative endeavors.

Understanding and Compassion: This gemstone enhances understanding and compassion, both towards oneself and others. It aids in seeing different perspectives and fosters empathetic relationships.

Positive Attitude: Yellow Aventurine promotes a positive, optimistic outlook on life. It helps overcome negativity and pessimism, encouraging a more joyful and enthusiastic approach to daily activities.

Emotional Balance: The stone aids in balancing emotions, reducing anxiety and stress. It encourages a feeling of inner peace and calm, helping to manage emotional responses more effectively.

Confidence and Self-Empowerment: Yellow Aventurine boosts self-confidence and empowerment. It assists individuals in taking control of their lives and making decisions that reflect their true desires.

Physical Healing Properties

Digestive Health: Associated with the solar plexus chakra, Yellow Aventurine is believed to aid in the digestive process and can help alleviate issues such as nausea and indigestion.

Immune System Support: This stone may enhance the immune system, providing a boost in overall health and protection against illness.

Detoxification: Yellow Aventurine supports the body's detoxification processes, aiding in the removal of toxins and promoting a healthier physical state.

Skin Health: It is also thought to benefit the skin, improving skin health and contributing to a clearer complexion.

Energy Levels: Yellow Aventurine can increase physical energy and vitality, reducing feelings of lethargy and fatigue.

Potential Homeopathic Uses

Psychological Symptoms: Addresses issues such as lack of creativity, difficulties in understanding others, and negative attitudes towards life.

Physical Symptoms: Supports digestive health, boosts the immune system, aids in detoxification, improves skin health, and enhances overall energy levels.

Behavioral Symptoms: Encourages a positive outlook, fosters emotional balance, and promotes self-confidence and empowerment.

Yellow Aventurine's homeopathic profile emphasizes its ability to inspire creativity, promote a positive outlook, and support physical health, making it suitable for a range of conditions related to emotional well-being and physical vitality.

Conclusion

Yellow Aventurine is a significant gemstone in holistic healing, appreciated not only for its beautiful appearance but also for its extensive healing properties. Whether used to enhance creative expression, foster a positive attitude, or support physical health, Yellow Aventurine serves as a powerful tool in achieving a balanced and fulfilling life. As with all alternative practices, these should be considered complementary to conventional medical treatments, integral to a holistic approach to health.

Yellow Calcite: Comprehensive Guide on Spiritual and Physical Healing Properties

Overview

Yellow Calcite, known for its bright, cheerful yellow color, is a crystal celebrated for its ability to stimulate the intellect, boost memory, and enhance learning abilities. This stone is particularly valued for its effectiveness in clearing mental clutter, facilitating a deeper understanding of the root causes of personal issues, and promoting a clear path to resolution.

Spiritual and Psychic Benefits

Intellectual Stimulation: Yellow Calcite activates the higher mind, enhancing intellectual efficiency and the capacity for critical thinking. It stimulates mental energy, making it easier to process and integrate new information.

Memory Enhancement: This gemstone is known for its ability to improve memory function, making it an excellent aid for students and professionals who need to retain large amounts of information.

Learning Abilities: Yellow Calcite enhances overall learning abilities, facilitating faster and more effective learning processes. It helps in understanding complex concepts and encourages a lifelong passion for discovery.

Clearing Mental Clutter: The stone is particularly effective in helping clear the mind of unnecessary thoughts and mental clutter. This clarity allows for a focused approach to problem-solving and decision-making.

Discovery of Problem Roots: By promoting mental clarity, Yellow Calcite aids in uncovering the underlying causes of various personal and professional issues, enabling a more strategic approach to challenges.

Physical Healing Properties

Energy Boost: Yellow Calcite invigorates the body, providing a boost to overall energy levels. This can be particularly beneficial during times of physical or mental fatigue.

Stress Reduction: The stone's calming effects on the mind also help reduce stress levels, promoting a state of relaxation and well-being.

Digestive Health: Yellow Calcite is said to support the digestive system, aiding in the improvement of metabolism and alleviation of digestive disorders.

Immune System Enhancement: It may also help strengthen the immune system, enhancing the body's ability to fight off infections and recover more quickly from illness.

Detoxification: Supporting the body's natural detoxification processes, Yellow Calcite helps in cleansing the liver and kidneys, promoting better health and vitality.

Potential Homeopathic Uses

Psychological Symptoms: Addresses issues such as poor concentration, difficulty in learning, memory lapses, and excessive mental clutter.

Physical Symptoms: Enhances energy levels, supports digestive health, boosts the immune system, and aids in stress relief and detoxification.

Behavioral Symptoms: Encourages a proactive approach to learning, improves focus and clarity in problem-solving, and fosters intellectual growth.

Yellow Calcite's homeopathic profile emphasizes its ability to stimulate intellectual and physical processes, making it suitable for a range of conditions related to mental performance, educational challenges, and overall physical health.

Conclusion

Yellow Calcite is a significant gemstone in holistic healing, appreciated not only for its vibrant appearance but also for its extensive intellectual and physical healing properties. Whether used to enhance mental capacities, support physical health, or foster clear and effective problem-solving, Yellow Calcite serves as a powerful tool in achieving a balanced and productive life. As with all alternative practices, these should be considered complementary to conventional medical treatments, integral to a holistic approach to health.

Yellow Opal: Comprehensive Guide on Spiritual and Physical Healing Properties

Overview

Yellow Opal, known for its translucent to opaque and vibrant yellow hue, is a stone deeply connected to emotional stability. It is celebrated for its ability to amplify positive emotions and infuse life with optimism and cheerfulness. This gemstone is particularly beneficial for those looking to enhance their emotional well-being and maintain a positive outlook on life.

Spiritual and Psychic Benefits

Emotional Stability: Yellow Opal helps stabilize emotions, providing a calming influence that can soothe erratic or tumultuous feelings. It assists in maintaining a balanced emotional state, which is crucial for overall well-being.

Amplification of Positive Emotions: This stone is known for its ability to enhance positive feelings such as joy, peace, and love. It encourages the expression and experience of positive emotions, contributing to a happier and more fulfilling life.

Optimism and Cheerfulness: Yellow Opal infuses its bearer with a sense of optimism and an uplifting energy. It helps dispel negativity and fosters a positive, cheerful attitude towards everyday situations.

Enhanced Emotional Expression: The gemstone facilitates clearer and more honest expression of emotions. It encourages open communication of feelings, aiding in relationship dynamics and personal growth.

Spiritual Connection: Yellow Opal can also enhance spiritual connections by aligning one's personal will with divine will, encouraging a deeper understanding of one's spiritual journey and purpose.

Physical Healing Properties

Digestive Health: Yellow Opal is believed to have a positive effect on the digestive system, aiding in better digestion and alleviating issues such as indigestion or heartburn.

Detoxification: This stone supports the body's detoxification processes, helping to cleanse the liver and kidneys and improve overall physical health.

Energizing: Yellow Opal can provide a gentle boost of energy, reducing feelings of lethargy and increasing stamina and vitality.

Immune System Support: It may also enhance the immune system, providing a general strengthening of the body's natural defenses against illness.

Skin Health: Yellow Opal is sometimes used to improve skin health, helping to brighten the complexion and treat minor skin irritations.

Potential Homeopathic Uses

Psychological Symptoms: Addresses issues like emotional instability, pessimism, negativity, and challenges in expressing emotions.

Physical Symptoms: Supports digestive health, aids in detoxification, boosts energy levels, enhances immune function, and assists in maintaining healthy skin.

Behavioral Symptoms: Encourages a more optimistic outlook, promotes the expression of positive emotions, and enhances overall cheerfulness and contentment.

Yellow Opal's homeopathic profile emphasizes its ability to stabilize and enhance emotional well-being, support physical health, and promote a positive, optimistic attitude, making it suitable for a range of conditions related to emotional health and physical vitality.

Conclusion

Yellow Opal is a valuable gemstone in holistic healing, appreciated not only for its beautiful appearance but also for its extensive healing properties. Whether used to foster emotional stability, enhance physical health, or cultivate a positive and cheerful outlook, Yellow Opal serves as a powerful tool in achieving a balanced and joyful life. As with all alternative practices, these should be considered complementary to conventional medical treatments, integral to a holistic approach to health.

Zebra Rock: Comprehensive Guide on Spiritual and Physical Healing Properties

Overview

Zebra Rock, characterized by its distinctive striped patterns reminiscent of a zebra's coat, is not only visually striking but also known for its healing properties. It is particularly valued for its ability to aid with skin ailments and enhance physical energy and stamina. This makes it an excellent choice for athletes or anyone engaged in physically demanding activities.

Spiritual and Psychic Benefits

Grounding: Zebra Rock is a grounding stone that helps stabilize and connect the physical body to the earth. This grounding effect is essential for maintaining a clear mind and focused energy, especially during intense physical activities.

Energy and Stamina: This stone is known for boosting physical energy and endurance, making it highly beneficial for athletes or individuals with active lifestyles. It provides the stamina needed for extended physical performance and helps in recovery.

Emotional Balance: Zebra Rock promotes emotional balance by helping to reduce anxiety and stress. Its calming properties aid in maintaining composure in challenging situations.

Mental Clarity: The grounding properties of Zebra Rock also enhance mental clarity. It assists in organizing thoughts and improving concentration, which is beneficial in both personal and professional settings.

Enhanced Motivation: By boosting energy levels and providing mental clarity, Zebra Rock also helps to enhance motivation, encouraging individuals to pursue and achieve their goals with persistence.

Physical Healing Properties

Skin Health: Zebra Rock is particularly noted for its ability to improve skin conditions. It helps in treating various skin ailments, promoting healthier skin and a more vibrant complexion.

Physical Recovery: The stone aids in the recovery process of the body, particularly after physical exertion or injury. It helps muscles relax and reduces inflammation, speeding up healing.

Enhanced Circulation: Zebra Rock can improve blood circulation, which in turn enhances energy distribution and health across the body, supporting overall vitality.

Detoxification: This stone supports the body's detoxification processes, aiding in the removal of toxins and promoting a healthier physical state.

Immune System Support: Zebra Rock may also contribute to strengthening the immune system, enhancing the body's ability to fight off infections and illnesses.

Potential Homeopathic Uses

Psychological Symptoms: Addresses issues such as lack of focus, low motivation, emotional instability, and stress-related mental fatigue.

Physical Symptoms: Supports skin health, aids in physical recovery and detoxification, enhances blood circulation, and boosts immune function.

Behavioral Symptoms: Encourages perseverance in physical activities, promotes balanced emotional reactions, and helps maintain high energy levels and stamina.

Zebra Rock's homeopathic profile emphasizes its ability to enhance physical stamina, support emotional and mental health, and promote overall physical healing, making it suitable for a range of conditions related to physical activity, skin health, and emotional balance.

Conclusion

Zebra Rock is a significant stone in holistic healing, appreciated not only for its unique appearance but also for its extensive healing properties. Whether used to support skin health, enhance physical stamina, or stabilize emotions, Zebra Rock serves as a potent tool in achieving a balanced and healthy life. As with all alternative practices, these should be considered complementary to conventional medical treatments, integral to a holistic approach to health.

Heliodor: Comprehensive Guide on Spiritual and Physical Healing Properties

Overview

Heliodor, known for its brilliant golden-yellow hues, is a captivating crystal cherished for its radiant energy and healing properties. This gemstone is often associated with sunlight and warmth, symbolizing vitality and mental clarity. Heliodor is celebrated for its ability to invigorate the spirit and promote overall well-being.

Spiritual and Psychic Benefits

Stress Relief and Calming: Heliodor is renowned for its ability to alleviate stress and anxiety. Its warm energy promotes a sense of peace and tranquility, helping to calm the mind and body. This makes it an excellent companion for meditation and relaxation practices.

Spiritual Growth: Connected to the solar plexus chakra, Heliodor enhances personal power and spiritual growth. It encourages self-confidence and clarity, helping individuals connect with their inner wisdom and purpose.

Protection: Heliodor acts as a protective shield against negative energies and emotional harm. It is particularly effective in safeguarding against stress and psychic attacks, creating a safe and nurturing environment for spiritual activities.

Enhancement of Healing Energies: Known for its ability to amplify healing energies, Heliodor is used to enhance both personal energy and the effectiveness of other healing crystals. It is beneficial in promoting a balanced and harmonious energy flow during crystal healing sessions.

Harmonization and Balance: Heliodor aids in balancing the body's subtle energies. It aligns the chakras and stabilizes emotions, fostering a harmonious internal environment that supports emotional well-being.

Versatile Use in Healing Practices: Utilized in various forms such as raw crystals, jewelry, and meditation tools, Heliodor is a key component in holistic healing practices. It is often used in energy layouts to align and balance the body's energy centers.

Physical Healing Properties

Vitality and Energy: Heliodor is believed to boost physical vitality and energy levels. It helps to invigorate the body, enhancing stamina and overall health.

Digestive Health: This crystal supports the digestive system, helping to alleviate issues such as indigestion and stomach discomfort. It promotes a healthy digestive process and aids in nutrient absorption.

Detoxification: Heliodor aids in detoxifying the body, supporting liver function and cleansing the system of toxins. This contributes to improved metabolic health and overall well-being.

Eye Health: Traditionally, Heliodor has been associated with eye health. It is believed to strengthen vision and protect against eye-related issues.

Cellular Regeneration: Heliodor supports the body's natural healing processes by promoting cellular regeneration. It aids in the recovery from injuries and illnesses, speeding up the healing process.

Potential Homeopathic Uses

Psychological Symptoms: Anxiety, low self-esteem, and mental fatigue. It may also help in cases of lack of clarity and focus.

Physical Symptoms: Digestive issues, low energy levels, and detoxification needs.

Behavioral Symptoms: Difficulty in coping with stress, lack of motivation, and a tendency towards emotional instability.

Heliodor's homeopathic profile would focus on its ability to invigorate, protect, and stabilize, making it suitable for addressing conditions related to stress, energy depletion, and digestive health.

Conclusion

Heliodor is a vital crystal in holistic healing, celebrated for its radiant beauty and versatile use in healing practices. Whether used to alleviate stress, enhance personal power, or support physical health,

Heliodor serves as a powerful tool in achieving a balanced and vibrant life. As with all alternative practices, these should be considered complementary to conventional medical treatments, forming an integral part of a holistic approach to health.

Scapolite: Comprehensive Guide on Spiritual and Physical Healing Properties

Overview

Scapolite, known for its range of colors from yellow to pink and violet, is a fascinating crystal prized for its clarity and transformative energy. This gemstone is often associated with problem-solving and personal growth. Scapolite is celebrated for its ability to enhance intellectual clarity and promote overall well-being.

Spiritual and Psychic Benefits

Stress Relief and Calming: Scapolite is renowned for its ability to reduce stress and anxiety. Its soothing energy fosters a sense of peace and tranquility, helping to calm the mind and alleviate mental tension. This makes it an excellent companion for relaxation and stress management.

Intellectual Clarity: Connected to the crown chakra, Scapolite enhances intellectual clarity and mental focus. It encourages clear thinking and problem-solving, helping individuals to approach challenges with a calm and rational mindset.

Emotional Resilience: Scapolite acts as a stabilizing force for emotions, aiding in the release of negative patterns and emotional blockages. It is particularly effective in promoting resilience and emotional strength, allowing for a balanced and harmonious emotional state.

Enhancement of Healing Energies: Known for its ability to amplify healing energies, Scapolite is used to enhance both personal energy and the effectiveness of other healing crystals. It is beneficial in promoting a balanced and harmonious energy flow during healing sessions.

Harmonization and Balance: Scapolite aids in balancing the body's subtle energies. It aligns the chakras and stabilizes emotions, fostering a harmonious internal environment that supports intellectual and emotional well-being.

Versatile Use in Healing Practices: Utilized in various forms such as raw crystals, jewelry, and meditation tools, Scapolite is a key component in holistic healing practices. It is often used in energy layouts to align and balance the body's energy centers.

Physical Healing Properties

Pain Relief: Scapolite is believed to support pain relief, especially for headaches and migraines. It helps to alleviate discomfort and promote overall well-being.

Eye Health: This crystal is traditionally associated with eye health. It is believed to strengthen vision and protect against eye-related issues, enhancing clarity and focus.

Digestive Health: Scapolite supports the digestive system, helping to alleviate issues such as indigestion and stomach discomfort. It promotes a healthy digestive process and aids in nutrient absorption.

Detoxification: Scapolite aids in detoxifying the body, supporting liver function and cleansing the system of toxins. This contributes to improved metabolic health and overall vitality.

Bone and Joint Health: Scapolite is believed to support bone and joint health, helping to strengthen bones and alleviate joint pain. It is beneficial for those dealing with arthritis and other joint-related issues.

Potential Homeopathic Uses

If Scapolite were to be used as a homeopathic remedy, its indications might include:

Psychological Symptoms: Mental fatigue, difficulty in concentration, and anxiety. It may also help in cases of emotional instability and stress.

Physical Symptoms: Headaches, eye strain, digestive issues, and detoxification needs.

Behavioral Symptoms: Difficulty in coping with intellectual stress, lack of focus, and a tendency towards emotional imbalance.

Scapolite's homeopathic profile would focus on its ability to clarify, soothe, and stabilize, making it suitable for addressing conditions related to intellectual clarity, stress management, and overall well-being.

Conclusion

Scapolite is a vital crystal in holistic healing, celebrated for its transformative clarity and versatile healing properties. Whether used for stress relief, intellectual enhancement, or as a stabilizing talisman, Scapolite serves as a potent aid in achieving physical health and spiritual harmony. Like all alternative practices, these should be considered as complementary to conventional medical treatments.

Larvikite: Comprehensive Guide on Spiritual and Physical Healing Properties

Overview

Larvikite, known for its striking blue and silver flashes, is a captivating crystal appreciated for its protective and grounding energy. This gemstone is often associated with earth connection and psychic abilities. Larvikite is celebrated for its ability to enhance intuition and promote overall well-being.

Spiritual and Psychic Benefits

Stress Relief and Calming: Larvikite is renowned for its ability to alleviate stress and anxiety. Its grounding energy promotes a sense of peace and stability, helping to calm the mind and body. This makes it an excellent companion for meditation and relaxation practices.

Intuition Enhancement: Connected to the third eye and root chakras, Larvikite enhances intuition and psychic abilities. It encourages clear thinking and spiritual insight, helping individuals to connect with their inner guidance and the natural world.

Protection: Larvikite acts as a protective shield against negative energies and psychic attacks. It is particularly effective in safeguarding against emotional and spiritual harm, creating a safe and nurturing environment for spiritual activities.

Enhancement of Healing Energies: Known for its ability to amplify healing energies, Larvikite is used to enhance both personal energy and the effectiveness of other healing crystals. It is beneficial in promoting a balanced and harmonious energy flow during healing sessions.

Harmonization and Balance: Larvikite aids in balancing the body's subtle energies. It aligns the chakras and stabilizes emotions, fostering a harmonious internal environment that supports emotional and spiritual well-being.

Versatile Use in Healing Practices: Utilized in various forms such as raw crystals, jewelry, and meditation tools, Larvikite is a key component in holistic healing practices. It is often used in energy layouts to align and balance the body's energy centers.

Physical Healing Properties

Vitality and Energy: Larvikite is believed to boost physical vitality and energy levels. It helps to invigorate the body, enhancing stamina and overall health.

Detoxification: Larvikite aids in detoxifying the body, supporting liver function and cleansing the system of toxins. This contributes to improved metabolic health and overall well-being.

Cognitive Function: Larvikite is associated with enhancing cognitive function. It supports mental clarity, focus, and decision-making, making it beneficial for those dealing with mental fatigue and confusion.

Immune System: Larvikite is believed to enhance the immune system, helping the body to fight off illnesses more effectively. It supports the body's natural defenses and promotes overall health and vitality.

Skin Health: Larvikite supports skin health by promoting cellular regeneration. It aids in the healing of skin conditions and improves the overall appearance of the skin.

Potential Homeopathic Uses

If Larvikite were to be used as a homeopathic remedy, its indications might include:

Psychological Symptoms: Anxiety, mental fatigue, and stress. It may also help in cases of emotional instability and lack of focus.

Physical Symptoms: Detoxification needs, immune system support, and skin conditions.

Behavioral Symptoms: Difficulty in coping with stress, lack of motivation, and a tendency towards emotional imbalance.

Larvikite's homeopathic profile would focus on its ability to ground, protect, and invigorate, making it suitable for addressing conditions related to stress, cognitive function, and overall well-being.

Conclusion

Larvikite is a vital crystal in holistic healing, celebrated for its grounding beauty and versatile healing properties. Whether used for stress relief, intuitive enhancement, or as a protective talisman, Larvikite serves as a potent aid in achieving physical health and spiritual harmony. Like all alternative practices, these should be considered as complementary to conventional medical treatments.

Chalcopyrite: Comprehensive Guide on Spiritual and Physical Healing Properties

Overview

Chalcopyrite, known for its vibrant metallic luster with hues of gold, green, and blue, is a striking crystal admired for its transformative energy and healing properties. This gemstone is often associated with abundance and joy. Chalcopyrite is celebrated for its ability to enhance perception and promote overall well-being.

Spiritual and Psychic Benefits

Stress Relief and Calming: Chalcopyrite is renowned for its ability to alleviate stress and anxiety. Its joyful energy promotes a sense of happiness and relaxation, helping to calm the mind and uplift the spirit. This makes it an excellent companion for stress management and emotional healing practices.

Spiritual Insight: Connected to the third eye and crown chakras, Chalcopyrite enhances spiritual insight and intuition. It encourages clear thinking and spiritual growth, helping individuals to connect with their inner wisdom and higher consciousness.

Abundance and Prosperity: Chalcopyrite is often associated with attracting abundance and prosperity. It is believed to manifest wealth and success, making it a popular crystal for those seeking financial growth and opportunities.

Enhancement of Healing Energies: Known for its ability to amplify healing energies, Chalcopyrite is used to enhance both personal energy and the effectiveness of other healing crystals. It is beneficial in promoting a balanced and harmonious energy flow during healing sessions.

Harmonization and Balance: Chalcopyrite aids in balancing the body's subtle energies. It aligns the chakras and stabilizes emotions, fostering a harmonious internal environment that supports emotional and spiritual well-being.

Versatile Use in Healing Practices: Utilized in various forms such as raw crystals, jewelry, and meditation tools, Chalcopyrite is a key component in holistic healing practices. It is often used in energy layouts to align and balance the body's energy centers.

Physical Healing Properties

Vitality and Energy: Chalcopyrite is believed to boost physical vitality and energy levels. It helps to invigorate the body, enhancing stamina and overall health.

Immune System: Chalcopyrite is believed to enhance the immune system, helping the body to fight off illnesses more effectively. It supports the body's natural defenses and promotes overall health and vitality.

Detoxification: Chalcopyrite aids in detoxifying the body, supporting liver function and cleansing the system of toxins. This contributes to improved metabolic health and overall well-being.

Inflammation Reduction: Chalcopyrite is associated with reducing inflammation and pain. It supports the body's natural healing processes, making it beneficial for those dealing with chronic pain and inflammatory conditions.

Cognitive Function: Chalcopyrite supports cognitive function by promoting mental clarity and focus. It is beneficial for those dealing with mental fatigue and confusion, enhancing overall cognitive performance.

Potential Homeopathic Uses

If Chalcopyrite were to be used as a homeopathic remedy, its indications might include:

Psychological Symptoms: Anxiety, emotional stress, and mental fatigue. It may also help in cases of lack of focus and clarity.

Physical Symptoms: Immune system deficiencies, detoxification needs, and inflammation.

Behavioral Symptoms: Difficulty in coping with stress, lack of motivation, and a tendency towards emotional imbalance.

Chalcopyrite's homeopathic profile would focus on its ability to invigorate, protect, and harmonize, making it suitable for addressing conditions related to stress, cognitive function, and overall well-being.

Conclusion

Chalcopyrite is a vital crystal in holistic healing, celebrated for its vibrant beauty and versatile healing properties. Whether used for stress relief, spiritual insight, or as a talisman for abundance, Chalcopyrite serves as a potent aid in achieving physical health and spiritual harmony. Like all alternative practices, these should be considered as complementary to conventional medical treatments.

Idocrase: Comprehensive Guide on Spiritual and Physical Healing Properties

Overview

Idocrase, also known as Vesuvianite, is a captivating crystal with colors ranging from green to brown. This gemstone is often associated with personal growth and transformation. Idocrase is celebrated for its ability to enhance mental clarity and promote overall well-being.

Spiritual and Psychic Benefits

Stress Relief and Calming: Idocrase is renowned for its ability to alleviate stress and anxiety. Its soothing energy promotes a sense of peace and tranquility, helping to calm the mind and body. This makes it an excellent companion for meditation and stress management practices.

Personal Growth: Connected to the heart and solar plexus chakras, Idocrase enhances personal growth and self-discovery. It encourages confidence and clarity, helping individuals to explore their true potential and purpose.

Transformation: Idocrase is a stone of transformation, aiding in the release of old patterns and the acceptance of new beginnings. It supports spiritual evolution and helps individuals navigate life changes with grace and resilience.

Enhancement of Healing Energies: Known for its ability to amplify healing energies, Idocrase is used to enhance both personal energy and the effectiveness of other healing crystals. It is beneficial in promoting a balanced and harmonious energy flow during healing sessions.

Harmonization and Balance: Idocrase aids in balancing the body's subtle energies. It aligns the chakras and stabilizes emotions, fostering a harmonious internal environment that supports emotional and spiritual well-being.

Versatile Use in Healing Practices: Utilized in various forms such as raw crystals, jewelry, and meditation tools, Idocrase is a key component

in holistic healing practices. It is often used in energy layouts to align and balance the body's energy centers.

Physical Healing Properties

Vitality and Energy: Idocrase is believed to boost physical vitality and energy levels. It helps to invigorate the body, enhancing stamina and overall health.

Digestive Health: This crystal supports the digestive system, helping to alleviate issues such as indigestion and stomach discomfort. It promotes a healthy digestive process and aids in nutrient absorption.

Detoxification: Idocrase aids in detoxifying the body, supporting liver function and cleansing the system of toxins. This contributes to improved metabolic health and overall well-being .

Cellular Regeneration: Idocrase supports the body's natural healing processes by promoting cellular regeneration. It aids in the recovery from injuries and illnesses, speeding up the healing process.

Bone and Joint Health: Idocrase is believed to support bone and joint health, helping to strengthen bones and alleviate joint pain. It is beneficial for those dealing with arthritis and other joint-related issues.

Potential Homeopathic Uses

If Idocrase were to be used as a homeopathic remedy, its indications might include:

Psychological Symptoms: Anxiety, emotional stress, and lack of clarity. It may also help in cases of emotional instability and indecision.

Physical Symptoms: Digestive health issues, detoxification needs, and joint pain.

Behavioral Symptoms: Difficulty in coping with stress, lack of motivation, and a tendency towards emotional imbalance.

Idocrase's homeopathic profile would focus on its ability to transform, clarify, and invigorate, making it suitable for addressing conditions related to stress, digestive health, and overall well-being.

Conclusion

Idocrase is a vital crystal in holistic healing, celebrated for its transformative beauty and versatile healing properties. Whether used for stress relief, personal growth, or as a talisman for transformation, Idocrase serves as a potent aid in achieving physical health and spiritual harmony. Like all alternative practices, these should be considered as complementary to conventional medical treatments.

Mookaite: Comprehensive Guide on Spiritual and Physical Healing Properties

Overview

Mookaite, also known as Mookaite Jasper, is a vibrant crystal with colors ranging from red and yellow to purple and brown. This gemstone is often associated with grounding and vitality. Mookaite is celebrated for its ability to enhance personal strength and promote overall well-being.

Spiritual and Psychic Benefits

Stress Relief and Calming: Mookaite is renowned for its ability to alleviate stress and anxiety. Its grounding energy promotes a sense of stability and balance, helping to calm the mind and body. This makes it an excellent companion for meditation and stress management practices.

Grounding and Stability: Connected to the root chakra, Mookaite enhances grounding and stability. It encourages a strong connection to the earth, helping individuals to feel secure and centered.

Personal Strength: Mookaite is a stone of personal strength and vitality. It supports self-confidence and courage, helping individuals to face challenges with determination and resilience.

Enhancement of Healing Energies: Known for its ability to amplify healing energies, Mookaite is used to enhance both personal energy and the effectiveness of other healing crystals. It is beneficial

in promoting a balanced and harmonious energy flow during healing sessions.

Harmonization and Balance: Mookaite aids in balancing the body's subtle energies. It aligns the chakras and stabilizes emotions, fostering a harmonious internal environment that supports emotional and physical well-being.

Versatile Use in Healing Practices: Utilized in various forms such as raw crystals, jewelry, and meditation tools, Mookaite is a key component in holistic healing practices. It is often used in energy layouts to align and balance the body's energy centers.

Physical Healing Properties

Vitality and Energy: Mookaite is believed to boost physical vitality and energy levels. It helps to invigorate the body, enhancing stamina and overall health.

Immune System: Mookaite is believed to enhance the immune system, helping the body to fight off illnesses more effectively. It supports the body's natural defenses and promotes overall health and vitality.

Digestive Health: This crystal supports the digestive system, helping to alleviate issues such as indigestion and stomach discomfort. It promotes a healthy digestive process and aids in nutrient absorption.

Detoxification: Mookaite aids in detoxifying the body, supporting liver function and cleansing the system of toxins. This contributes to improved metabolic health and overall well-being.

Healing and Regeneration: Mookaite supports the body's natural healing processes by promoting cellular regeneration. It aids in the recovery from injuries and illnesses, speeding up the healing process.

Potential Homeopathic Uses

If Mookaite were to be used as a homeopathic remedy, its indications might include:

Psychological Symptoms: Anxiety, stress, and lack of confidence. It may also help in cases of emotional instability and lack of motivation.

Physical Symptoms: Digestive health issues, immune system deficiencies, and detoxification needs.

Behavioral Symptoms: Difficulty in coping with stress, lack of resilience, and a tendency towards emotional imbalance.

Mookaite's homeopathic profile would focus on its ability to ground, invigorate, and stabilize, making it suitable for addressing conditions related to stress, digestive health, and overall well-being.

Conclusion

Mookaite is a vital crystal in holistic healing, celebrated for its vibrant beauty and versatile healing properties. Whether used for stress relief, personal strength, or as a grounding talisman, Mookaite serves as a potent aid in achieving physical health and spiritual harmony. Like all alternative practices, these should be considered as complementary to conventional medical treatments.

Brookite: Comprehensive Guide on Spiritual and Physical Healing Properties

Overview

Brookite, known for its striking brown to black hues with shimmering inclusions, is a rare crystal valued for its high-frequency energy and transformative properties. This gemstone is often associated with spiritual awakening and clarity. Brookite is celebrated for its ability to elevate consciousness and promote overall well-being.

Spiritual and Psychic Benefits

Stress Relief and Calming: Brookite is renowned for its ability to alleviate stress and anxiety. Its high-frequency energy promotes a sense of calm and tranquility, helping to clear the mind and reduce emotional tension. This makes it an excellent companion for meditation and spiritual practices.

Spiritual Awakening: Connected to the crown and third eye chakras, Brookite enhances spiritual awakening and higher consciousness. It encourages clarity of thought and spiritual insight, helping individuals to connect with their higher self and the universe.

Transformation and Growth: Brookite is a stone of transformation, aiding in personal and spiritual growth. It supports the release of old patterns and the acceptance of new perspectives, facilitating profound changes in one's life.

Enhancement of Healing Energies: Known for its ability to amplify healing energies, Brookite is used to enhance both personal energy and the effectiveness of other healing crystals. It is beneficial in promoting a balanced and harmonious energy flow during healing sessions.

Harmonization and Balance: Brookite aids in balancing the body's subtle energies. It aligns the chakras and stabilizes emotions, fostering a harmonious internal environment that supports spiritual and emotional well-being.

Versatile Use in Healing Practices: Utilized in various forms such as raw crystals, jewelry, and meditation tools, Brookite is a key component in holistic healing practices
. It is often used in energy layouts to align and balance the body's energy centers.

Physical Healing Properties

Vitality and Energy: Brookite is believed to boost physical vitality and energy levels. It helps to invigorate the body, enhancing stamina and overall health.

Detoxification: Brookite aids in detoxifying the body, supporting liver function and cleansing the system of toxins. This contributes to improved metabolic health and overall well-being.

Cellular Regeneration: Brookite supports the body's natural healing processes by promoting cellular regeneration. It aids in the recovery from injuries and illnesses, speeding up the healing process.

Immune System: Brookite is believed to enhance the immune system, helping the body to fight off illnesses more effectively. It

supports the body's natural defenses and promotes overall health and vitality.

Bone and Joint Health: Brookite supports bone and joint health, helping to strengthen bones and alleviate joint pain. It is beneficial for those dealing with arthritis and other joint-related issues.

Potential Homeopathic Uses

If Brookite were to be used as a homeopathic remedy, its indications might include:

Psychological Symptoms: Anxiety, mental fatigue, and lack of clarity. It may also help in cases of emotional instability and spiritual confusion.

Physical Symptoms: Detoxification needs, immune system deficiencies, and joint pain.

Behavioral Symptoms: Difficulty in coping with stress, lack of motivation, and a tendency towards emotional imbalance.

Brookite's homeopathic profile would focus on its ability to transform, clarify, and invigorate, making it suitable for addressing conditions related to stress, detoxification, and overall well-being.

Conclusion

Brookite is a vital crystal in holistic healing, celebrated for its high-frequency energy and versatile healing properties. Whether used for stress relief, spiritual awakening, or as a transformative talisman, Brookite serves as a potent aid in achieving physical health and spiritual harmony. Like all alternative practices, these should be considered as complementary to conventional medical treatments.

Clinozoisite: Comprehensive Guide on Spiritual and Physical Healing Properties

Overview

Clinozoisite, known for its green to brownish hues and crystalline structure, is a fascinating crystal valued for its harmonizing and restorative energy. This gemstone is often associated with emotional healing and resilience. Clinozoisite is celebrated for its ability to enhance emotional stability and promote overall well-being.

Spiritual and Psychic Benefits

Stress Relief and Calming: Clinozoisite is renowned for its ability to alleviate stress and anxiety. Its soothing energy promotes a sense of peace and balance, helping to calm the mind and body. This makes it an excellent companion for meditation and stress management practices.

Emotional Healing: Connected to the heart chakra, Clinozoisite enhances emotional healing and resilience. It encourages the release of negative emotions and supports the healing of emotional wounds, helping individuals to achieve emotional balance and harmony.

Personal Growth: Clinozoisite supports personal growth and self-discovery. It encourages introspection and self-awareness, helping individuals to understand and overcome personal challenges.

Enhancement of Healing Energies: Known for its ability to amplify healing energies, Clinozoisite is used to enhance both personal energy and the effectiveness of other healing crystals. It is beneficial in promoting a balanced and harmonious energy flow during healing sessions.

Harmonization and Balance: Clinozoisite aids in balancing the body's subtle energies. It aligns the chakras and stabilizes emotions, fostering a harmonious internal environment that supports emotional and physical well-being.

Versatile Use in Healing Practices: Utilized in various forms such as raw crystals, jewelry, and meditation tools, Clinozoisite is a key component in holistic healing practices. It is often used in energy layouts to align and balance the body's energy centers.

Physical Healing Properties

Vitality and Energy: Clinozoisite is believed to boost physical vitality and energy levels. It helps to invigorate the body, enhancing stamina and overall health.

Bone and Joint Health: Clinozoisite supports bone and joint health, helping to strengthen bones and alleviate joint pain. It is beneficial for those dealing with arthritis and other joint-related issues.

Detoxification: Clinozoisite aids in detoxifying the body, supporting liver function and cleansing the system of toxins. This contributes to improved metabolic health and overall well-being.

Cellular Regeneration: Clinozoisite supports the body's natural healing processes by promoting cellular regeneration. It aids in the recovery from injuries and illnesses, speeding up the healing process.

Immune System: Clinozoisite is believed to enhance the immune system, helping the body to fight off illnesses more effectively. It supports the body's natural defenses and promotes overall health and vitality.

Potential Homeopathic Uses

If Clinozoisite were to be used as a homeopathic remedy, its indications might include:

Psychological Symptoms: Anxiety, emotional stress, and lack of clarity. It may also help in cases of emotional instability and vulnerability.

Physical Symptoms: Bone and joint health issues, detoxification needs, and energy depletion.

Behavioral Symptoms: Difficulty in coping with stress, lack of motivation, and a tendency towards emotional imbalance.

Clinozoisite's homeopathic profile would focus on its ability to heal, protect, and stabilize, making it suitable for addressing conditions related to stress, bone health, and overall well-being.

Conclusion

Clinozoisite is a vital crystal in holistic healing, celebrated for its harmonizing beauty and versatile healing properties. Whether used for stress relief, emotional healing, or as a restorative talisman, Clinozoisite serves as a potent aid in achieving physical health and spiritual harmony. Like all alternative practices, these should be considered as complementary to conventional medical treatments.

Covellite: Comprehensive Guide on Spiritual and Physical Healing Properties

Overview

Covellite, known for its deep blue and metallic sheen, is a captivating crystal cherished for its transformative and metaphysical properties. This gemstone is often associated with deep insight and spiritual evolution. Covellite is celebrated for its ability to enhance psychic abilities and promote overall well-being.

Spiritual and Psychic Benefits

Stress Relief and Calming: Covellite is renowned for its ability to alleviate stress and anxiety. Its calming energy promotes a sense of peace and tranquility, helping to clear the mind and reduce emotional tension. This makes it an excellent companion for meditation and spiritual practices.

Psychic Abilities: Connected to the third eye and crown chakras, Covellite enhances psychic abilities and intuition. It encourages deep insight and spiritual clarity, helping individuals to connect with their higher self and the metaphysical realm.

Spiritual Evolution: Covellite is a stone of transformation and spiritual evolution. It aids in the release of old patterns and the acceptance of new perspectives, facilitating profound changes in one's spiritual journey.

Enhancement of Healing Energies: Known for its ability to amplify healing energies, Covellite is used to enhance both personal energy and the effectiveness of other healing crystals. It is beneficial in promoting a balanced and harmonious energy flow during healing sessions.

Harmonization and Balance: Covellite aids in balancing the body's subtle energies. It aligns the chakras and stabilizes emotions, fostering a harmonious internal environment that supports spiritual and emotional well-being.

Versatile Use in Healing Practices: Utilized in various forms such as raw crystals, jewelry, and meditation tools, Covellite is a key component in holistic healing practices. It is often used in energy layouts to align and balance the body's energy centers.

Physical Healing Properties

Vitality and Energy: Covellite is believed to boost physical vitality and energy levels. It helps to invigorate the body, enhancing stamina and overall health.

Detoxification: Covellite aids in detoxifying the body, supporting liver function and cleansing the system of toxins. This contributes to improved metabolic health and overall well-being.

Cellular Regeneration: Covellite supports the body's natural healing processes by promoting cellular regeneration. It aids in the recovery from injuries and illnesses, speeding up the healing process.

Immune System: Covellite is believed to enhance the immune system, helping the body to fight off illnesses more effectively. It supports the body's natural defenses and promotes overall health and vitality.

Skin Health: Covellite supports skin health by promoting cellular regeneration and healing. It aids in the treatment of skin conditions and improves the overall appearance of the skin.

Potential Homeopathic Uses

If Covellite were to be used as a homeopathic remedy, its indications might include:

Psychological Symptoms: Anxiety, emotional stress, and lack of clarity. It may also help in cases of emotional instability and spiritual confusion.

Physical Symptoms: Detoxification needs, immune system deficiencies, and skin conditions.

Behavioral Symptoms: Difficulty in coping with stress, lack of motivation, and a tendency towards emotional imbalance.

Covellite's homeopathic profile would focus on its ability to transform, clarify, and rejuvenate, making it suitable for addressing conditions related to stress, detoxification, and overall well-being.

Conclusion

Covellite is a vital crystal in holistic healing, celebrated for its deep beauty and versatile healing properties. Whether used for stress relief, psychic enhancement, or as a transformative talisman, Covellite serves as a potent aid in achieving physical health and spiritual harmony. Like all alternative practices, these should be considered as complementary to conventional medical treatments.

Eilat Stone: Comprehensive Guide on Spiritual and Physical Healing Properties

Overview

Eilat Stone, known for its vibrant mix of blue, green, and turquoise colors, is a unique crystal valued for its rich mineral composition and healing energy. This gemstone is often associated with balance and harmony. Eilat Stone is celebrated for its ability to enhance emotional and physical well-being.

Spiritual and Psychic Benefits

Stress Relief and Calming: Eilat Stone is renowned for its ability to alleviate stress and anxiety. Its soothing energy promotes a sense of peace and relaxation, helping to calm the mind and body. This makes it an excellent companion for meditation and stress management practices.

Emotional Balance: Connected to the heart and throat chakras, Eilat Stone enhances emotional balance and communication. It encourages emotional healing and helps individuals express their feelings more effectively.

Harmony and Integration: Eilat Stone is a stone of balance and integration. It aids in harmonizing different aspects of oneself, promoting a sense of unity and wholeness. This supports personal growth and self-acceptance.

Enhancement of Healing Energies: Known for its ability to amplify healing energies, Eilat Stone is used to enhance both personal energy and the effectiveness of other healing crystals. It is beneficial in promoting a balanced and harmonious energy flow during healing sessions.

Harmonization and Balance: Eilat Stone aids in balancing the body's subtle energies. It aligns the chakras and stabilizes emotions, fostering a harmonious internal environment that supports emotional and physical well-being.

Versatile Use in Healing Practices: Utilized in various forms such as raw crystals, jewelry, and meditation tools, Eilat Stone is a key component in holistic healing practices. It is often used in energy layouts to align and balance the body's energy centers.

Physical Healing Properties

Vitality and Energy: Eilat Stone is believed to boost physical vitality and energy levels. It helps to invigorate the body, enhancing stamina and overall health.

Immune System: Eilat Stone is believed to enhance the immune system, helping the body to fight off illnesses more effectively. It supports the body's natural defenses and promotes overall health and vitality.

Pain Relief: This crystal supports pain relief, especially for joint and muscle pain. It helps to alleviate discomfort and promote overall well-being.

Detoxification: Eilat Stone aids in detoxifying the body, supporting liver function and cleansing the system of toxins. This contributes to improved metabolic health and overall well-being.

Healing and Regeneration: Eilat Stone supports the body's natural healing processes by promoting cellular regeneration. It aids in the recovery from injuries and illnesses, speeding up the healing process.

Potential Homeopathic Uses

If Eilat Stone were to be used as a homeopathic remedy, its indications might include:

Psychological Symptoms: Anxiety, emotional stress, and lack of clarity. It may also help in cases of emotional instability and difficulty in communication.

Physical Symptoms: Immune system deficiencies, detoxification needs, and joint pain.

Behavioral Symptoms: Difficulty in coping with stress, lack of motivation, and a tendency towards emotional imbalance.

Eilat Stone's homeopathic profile would focus on its ability to balance, protect, and rejuvenate, making it suitable for addressing conditions related to stress, immune health, and overall well-being.

Conclusion

Eilat Stone is a vital crystal in holistic healing, celebrated for its vibrant beauty and versatile healing properties. Whether used for stress relief, emotional balance, or as a harmonizing talisman, Eilat Stone serves as a potent aid in achieving physical health and spiritual harmony. Like all alternative practices, these should be considered as complementary to conventional medical treatments.

Galaxite: Comprehensive Guide on Spiritual and Physical Healing Properties

Overview

Galaxite, known for its shimmering, dark blue-black appearance with flashes of iridescent colors, is a mystical crystal valued for its cosmic energy and transformative properties. This gemstone is often associated with spiritual growth and protection. Galaxite is celebrated for its ability to enhance intuition and promote overall well-being.

Spiritual and Psychic Benefits

Stress Relief and Calming: Galaxite is renowned for its ability to alleviate stress and anxiety. Its calming energy promotes a sense of peace and tranquility, helping to soothe the mind and body. This makes it an excellent companion for meditation and spiritual practices.

Intuition and Psychic Abilities: Connected to the third eye and crown chakras, Galaxite enhances intuition and psychic abilities. It encourages spiritual insight and clarity, helping individuals to connect with their higher self and the universe.

Spiritual Growth: Galaxite is a stone of spiritual growth and evolution. It supports the release of old patterns and facilitates the acceptance of new perspectives, aiding in profound personal transformation.

Enhancement of Healing Energies: Known for its ability to amplify healing energies, Galaxite is used to enhance both personal energy and the effectiveness of other healing crystals. It is beneficial in promoting a balanced and harmonious energy flow during healing sessions.

Harmonization and Balance: Galaxite aids in balancing the body's subtle energies. It aligns the chakras and stabilizes emotions, fostering a harmonious internal environment that supports spiritual and emotional well-being.

Versatile Use in Healing Practices: Utilized in various forms such as raw crystals, jewelry, and meditation tools, Galaxite is a key component in holistic healing practices. It is often used in energy layouts to align and balance the body's energy centers.

Physical Healing Properties

Vitality and Energy: Galaxite is believed to boost physical vitality and energy levels. It helps to invigorate the body, enhancing stamina and overall health.

Detoxification: Galaxite aids in detoxifying the body, supporting liver function and cleansing the system of toxins. This contributes to improved metabolic health and overall well-being.

Immune System: Galaxite is believed to enhance the immune system, helping the body to fight off illnesses more effectively. It supports the body's natural defenses and promotes overall health and vitality.

Cellular Regeneration: Galaxite supports the body's natural healing processes by promoting cellular regeneration. It aids in the recovery from injuries and illnesses, speeding up the healing process.

Skin Health: Galaxite supports skin health by promoting cellular regeneration and healing. It aids in the treatment of skin conditions and improves the overall appearance of the skin.

Potential Homeopathic Uses

If Galaxite were to be used as a homeopathic remedy, its indications might include:

Psychological Symptoms: Anxiety, emotional stress, and lack of clarity. It may also help in cases of emotional instability and spiritual confusion.

Physical Symptoms: Detoxification needs, immune system deficiencies, and skin conditions.

Behavioral Symptoms: Difficulty in coping with stress, lack of motivation, and a tendency towards emotional imbalance.

Galaxite's homeopathic profile would focus on its ability to transform, protect, and rejuvenate, making it suitable for addressing conditions related to stress, detoxification, and overall well-being.

Conclusion

Galaxite is a vital crystal in holistic healing, celebrated for its mystical beauty and versatile healing properties. Whether used for stress relief, spiritual growth, or as a transformative talisman, Galaxite serves as a potent aid in achieving physical health and spiritual harmony. Like all alternative practices, these should be considered as complementary to conventional medical treatments.

Proustite: Comprehensive Guide on Spiritual and Physical Healing Properties

Overview

Proustite, known for its vibrant red to scarlet hues and striking crystal formations, is a rare and captivating crystal valued for its powerful energy and metaphysical properties. This gemstone is often associated with clarity and vitality. Proustite is celebrated for its ability to enhance intuition and promote overall well-being.

Spiritual and Psychic Benefits

Stress Relief and Calming: Proustite is renowned for its ability to alleviate stress and anxiety. Its vibrant energy promotes a sense of peace and tranquility, helping to calm the mind and reduce emotional tension. This makes it an excellent companion for meditation and stress management practices.

Intuition and Psychic Abilities: Connected to the root and third eye chakras, Proustite enhances intuition and psychic abilities. It encourages deep spiritual insight and clarity, helping individuals to connect with their inner wisdom and higher consciousness.

Vitality and Energy: Proustite is a stone of vitality and energy. It supports physical and emotional resilience, helping individuals to overcome fatigue and regain their strength.

Enhancement of Healing Energies: Known for its ability to amplify healing energies, Proustite is used to enhance both personal energy and the effectiveness of other healing crystals. It is beneficial in promoting a balanced and harmonious energy flow during healing sessions.

Harmonization and Balance: Proustite aids in balancing the body's subtle energies. It aligns the chakras and stabilizes emotions, fostering a harmonious internal environment that supports spiritual and emotional well-being.

Versatile Use in Healing Practices: Utilized in various forms such as raw crystals, jewelry, and meditation tools, Proustite is a key component in holistic healing practices. It is often used in energy layouts to align and balance the body's energy centers.

Physical Healing Properties

Vitality and Energy: Proustite is believed to boost physical vitality and energy levels. It helps to invigorate the body, enhancing stamina and overall health.

Blood Health: This crystal supports healthy blood circulation and detoxification. It helps to purify the blood and strengthen the cardiovascular system, contributing to overall vitality and well-being.

Detoxification: Proustite aids in detoxifying the body, supporting liver function and cleansing the system of toxins. This contributes to improved metabolic health and overall well-being.

Cellular Regeneration: Proustite supports the body's natural healing processes by promoting cellular regeneration. It aids in the recovery from injuries and illnesses, speeding up the healing process.

Immune System: Proustite is believed to enhance the immune system, helping the body to fight off illnesses more effectively. It supports the body's natural defenses and promotes overall health and vitality.

Potential Homeopathic Uses

If Proustite were to be used as a homeopathic remedy, its indications might include:

Psychological Symptoms: Anxiety, emotional stress, and lack of clarity. It may also help in cases of emotional instability and spiritual confusion.

Physical Symptoms: Blood health issues, detoxification needs, and immune system deficiencies.

Behavioral Symptoms: Difficulty in coping with stress, lack of motivation, and a tendency towards emotional imbalance.

Proustite's homeopathic profile would focus on its ability to invigorate, protect, and rejuvenate, making it suitable for addressing conditions related to stress, blood health, and overall well-being.

Conclusion

Proustite is a vital crystal in holistic healing, celebrated for its vibrant beauty and versatile healing properties. Whether used for stress relief, intuitive enhancement, or as a revitalizing talisman, Proustite serves as a potent aid in achieving physical health and spiritual harmony. Like all alternative practices, these should be considered as complementary to conventional medical treatments.

Spessartine: Comprehensive Guide on Spiritual and Physical Healing Properties

Overview

Spessartine, also known as Spessartine, is a variety of garnet known for its stunning orange to reddish-orange hues. This vibrant crystal is valued for its energizing and revitalizing properties. Spessartine is celebrated for its ability to enhance creativity and promote overall well-being.

Spiritual and Psychic Benefits

Stress Relief and Calming: Spessartine is renowned for its ability to alleviate stress and anxiety. Its invigorating energy promotes a sense of joy and enthusiasm, helping to uplift the spirit and dispel negative emotions. This makes it an excellent companion for meditation and stress management practices.

Creativity and Passion: Connected to the sacral chakra, Spessartine enhances creativity and passion. It encourages self-expression and inspires new ideas, making it a powerful tool for artists and creators.

Courage and Confidence: Spessartine is a stone of courage and confidence. It supports personal empowerment and resilience, helping individuals to face challenges with determination and optimism.

Enhancement of Healing Energies: Known for its ability to amplify healing energies, Spessartine is used to enhance both personal energy and the effectiveness of other healing crystals. It is beneficial in promoting a balanced and harmonious energy flow during healing sessions.

Harmonization and Balance: Spessartine aids in balancing the body's subtle energies. It aligns the chakras and stabilizes emotions, fostering a harmonious internal environment that supports emotional and physical well-being.

Versatile Use in Healing Practices: Utilized in various forms such as raw crystals, jewelry, and meditation tools, Spessartine is a key component in holistic healing practices. It is often used in energy layouts to align and balance the body's energy centers.

Physical Healing Properties

Vitality and Energy: Spessartine is believed to boost physical vitality and energy levels. It helps to invigorate the body, enhancing stamina and overall health.

Metabolism and Digestion: This crystal supports healthy metabolism and digestion. It helps to regulate the digestive system and alleviate issues such as indigestion and stomach discomfort.

Immune System: Spessartine is believed to enhance the immune system, helping the body to fight off illnesses more effectively. It supports the body's natural defenses and promotes overall health and vitality.

Detoxification: Spessartine aids in detoxifying the body, supporting liver function and cleansing the system of toxins. This contributes to improved metabolic health and overall well-being.

Healing and Regeneration: Spessartine supports the body's natural healing processes by promoting cellular regeneration. It aids in the recovery from injuries and illnesses, speeding up the healing process.

Potential Homeopathic Uses

If Spessartine were to be used as a homeopathic remedy, its indications might include:

Psychological Symptoms: Anxiety, low self-esteem, and lack of motivation. It may also help in cases of emotional instability and fear.

Physical Symptoms: Digestive health issues, immune system deficiencies, and detoxification needs.

Behavioral Symptoms: Difficulty in coping with stress, lack of creativity, and a tendency towards emotional imbalance.

Spessartine's homeopathic profile would focus on its ability to invigorate, protect, and inspire, making it suitable for addressing conditions related to stress, digestive health, and overall well-being.

Conclusion

Spessartine is a vital crystal in holistic healing, celebrated for its vibrant beauty and versatile healing properties. Whether used for stress relief, personal empowerment, or as a creative talisman, Spessartine serves as a potent aid in achieving physical health and spiritual harmony. Like all alternative practices, these should be considered as complementary to conventional medical treatments.

Cerussite: Comprehensive Guide on Spiritual and Physical Healing Properties

Overview

Cerussite, known for its clear to white crystalline appearance, is a unique crystal valued for its grounding and transformative energy. This gemstone is often associated with clarity and adaptability. Cerussite is celebrated for its ability to enhance mental clarity and promote overall well-being.

Spiritual and Psychic Benefits

Stress Relief and Calming: Cerussite is renowned for its ability to alleviate stress and anxiety. Its grounding energy promotes a sense of stability and calm, helping to clear the mind and reduce emotional tension. This makes it an excellent companion for meditation and stress management practices.

Mental Clarity: Connected to the root and crown chakras, Cerussite enhances mental clarity and focus. It encourages clear thinking and decision-making, helping individuals to approach challenges with confidence and determination.

Adaptability and Transformation: Cerussite is a stone of adaptability and transformation. It supports personal growth and resilience, helping individuals to navigate life changes with grace and ease.

Enhancement of Healing Energies: Known for its ability to amplify healing energies, Cerussite is used to enhance both personal energy and the effectiveness of other healing crystals. It is beneficial in promoting a balanced and harmonious energy flow during healing sessions.

Harmonization and Balance: Cerussite aids in balancing the body's subtle energies. It aligns the chakras and stabilizes emotions, fostering a harmonious internal environment that supports emotional and physical well-being.

Versatile Use in Healing Practices: Utilized in various forms such as raw crystals, jewelry, and meditation tools, Cerussite is a key component in holistic healing practices. It is often used in energy layouts to align and balance the body's energy centers.

Physical Healing Properties

Vitality and Energy: Cerussite is believed to boost physical vitality and energy levels. It helps to invigorate the body, enhancing stamina and overall health.

Bone and Joint Health: Cerussite supports bone and joint health, helping to strengthen bones and alleviate joint pain. It is beneficial for those dealing with arthritis and other joint-related issues.

Detoxification: Cerussite aids in detoxifying the body, supporting liver function and cleansing the system of toxins. This contributes to improved metabolic health and overall well-being.

Cellular Regeneration: Cerussite supports the body's natural healing processes by promoting cellular regeneration. It aids in the recovery from injuries and illnesses, speeding up the healing process.

Immune System: Cerussite is believed to enhance the immune system, helping the body to fight off illnesses more effectively. It supports the body's natural defenses and promotes overall health and vitality.

Potential Homeopathic Uses

If Cerussite were to be used as a homeopathic remedy, its indications might include:

Psychological Symptoms: Anxiety, emotional stress, and lack of clarity. It may also help in cases of emotional instability and difficulty adapting to change.

Physical Symptoms: Bone and joint health issues, detoxification needs, and immune system deficiencies.

Behavioral Symptoms: Difficulty in coping with stress, lack of motivation, and a tendency towards emotional imbalance.

Cerussite's homeopathic profile would focus on its ability to ground, protect, and transform, making it suitable for addressing conditions related to stress, bone health, and overall well-being.

Conclusion

Cerussite is a vital crystal in holistic healing, celebrated for its grounding beauty and versatile healing properties. Whether used for stress relief, mental clarity, or as a transformative talisman, Cerussite serves as a potent aid in achieving physical health and spiritual harmony. Like all alternative practices, these should be considered as complementary to conventional medical treatments.

Crocoite: Comprehensive Guide on Spiritual and Physical Healing Properties

Overview

Crocoite, known for its striking bright orange to red crystalline structure, is a rare and powerful crystal valued for its energizing and transformative properties. This gemstone is often associated with passion and vitality. Crocoite is celebrated for its ability to enhance creativity and promote overall well-being.

Spiritual and Psychic Benefits

Stress Relief and Calming: Crocoite is renowned for its ability to alleviate stress and anxiety. Its vibrant energy promotes a sense of joy and enthusiasm, helping to uplift the spirit and dispel negative emotions. This makes it an excellent companion for meditation and stress management practices.

Creativity and Passion: Connected to the sacral chakra, Crocoite enhances creativity and passion. It encourages self-expression and inspires new ideas, making it a powerful tool for artists and creators.

Transformation and Growth: Crocoite is a stone of transformation and growth. It supports the release of old patterns and the acceptance of new perspectives, facilitating profound changes in one's personal and spiritual journey.

Enhancement of Healing Energies: Known for its ability to amplify healing energies, Crocoite is used to enhance both personal energy and the effectiveness of other healing crystals. It is beneficial in promoting a balanced and harmonious energy flow during healing sessions.

Harmonization and Balance: Crocoite aids in balancing the body's subtle energies. It aligns the chakras and stabilizes emotions, fostering a harmonious internal environment that supports emotional and physical well-being.

Versatile Use in Healing Practices: Utilized in various forms such as raw crystals, jewelry, and meditation tools, Crocoite is a key component in holistic healing practices. It is often used in energy layouts to align and balance the body's energy centers.

Physical Healing Properties

Vitality and Energy: Crocoite is believed to boost physical vitality and energy levels. It helps to invigorate the body, enhancing stamina and overall health.

Detoxification: Crocoite aids in detoxifying the body, supporting liver function and cleansing the system of toxins. This contributes to improved metabolic health and overall well-being.

Immune System: Crocoite is believed to enhance the immune system, helping the body to fight off illnesses more effectively. It

supports the body's natural defenses and promotes overall health and vitality.

Reproductive Health: Crocoite supports reproductive health, helping to balance hormonal levels and enhance fertility. It is beneficial for those dealing with reproductive issues.

Healing and Regeneration: Crocoite supports the body's natural healing processes by promoting cellular regeneration. It aids in the recovery from injuries and illnesses, speeding up the healing process.

Potential Homeopathic Uses

If Crocoite were to be used as a homeopathic remedy, its indications might include:

Psychological Symptoms: Anxiety, emotional stress, and lack of clarity. It may also help in cases of emotional instability and difficulty focusing.

Physical Symptoms: Detoxification needs, immune system deficiencies, and joint pain.

Behavioral Symptoms: Difficulty in coping with stress, lack of motivation, and a tendency towards emotional imbalance.

Crocoite's homeopathic profile would focus on its ability to invigorate, transform, and inspire, making it suitable for addressing conditions related to stress, immune health, and overall well-being.

Conclusion

Crocoite is a vital crystal in holistic healing, celebrated for its vibrant beauty and versatile healing properties. Whether used for stress relief, personal empowerment, or as a transformative talisman, Crocoite serves as a potent aid in achieving physical health and spiritual harmony. Like all alternative practices, these should be considered as complementary to conventional medical treatments.

Hematite: Comprehensive Guide on Spiritual and Physical Healing Properties

Overview

Hematite, known for its metallic sheen and grounding energy, is a powerful crystal valued for its stabilizing and protective properties. This gemstone is often associated with strength and clarity. Hematite is celebrated for its ability to enhance focus and promote overall well-being.

Spiritual and Psychic Benefits

Stress Relief and Calming: Hematite is renowned for its ability to alleviate stress and anxiety. Its grounding energy promotes a sense of stability and calm, helping to clear the mind and reduce emotional tension. This makes it an excellent companion for meditation and stress management practices.

Grounding and Protection: Connected to the root chakra, Hematite enhances grounding and protection. It encourages a strong connection to the earth, helping individuals to feel secure and centered.

Mental Clarity: Hematite is a stone of mental clarity and focus. It supports clear thinking and decision-making, helping individuals to approach challenges with confidence and determination.

Enhancement of Healing Energies: Known for its ability to amplify healing energies, Hematite is used to enhance both personal energy and the effectiveness of other healing crystals. It is beneficial in promoting a balanced and harmonious energy flow during healing sessions.

Harmonization and Balance: Hematite aids in balancing the body's subtle energies. It aligns the chakras and stabilizes emotions, fostering a harmonious internal environment that supports emotional and physical well-being.

Versatile Use in Healing Practices: Utilized in various forms such as raw crystals, jewelry, and meditation tools, Hematite is a key component in holistic healing practices. It is often used in energy layouts to align and balance the body's energy centers.

Physical Healing Properties

Vitality and Energy: Hematite is believed to boost physical vitality and energy levels. It helps to invigorate the body, enhancing stamina and overall health.

Blood Health: This crystal supports healthy blood circulation and detoxification. It helps to purify the blood and strengthen the cardiovascular system, contributing to overall vitality and well-being.

Immune System: Hematite is believed to enhance the immune system, helping the body to fight off illnesses more effectively. It supports the body's natural defenses and promotes overall health and vitality.

Detoxification: Hematite aids in detoxifying the body, supporting liver function and cleansing the system of toxins. This contributes to improved metabolic health and overall well-being.

Bone and Joint Health: Hematite supports bone and joint health, helping to strengthen bones and alleviate joint pain. It is beneficial for those dealing with arthritis and other joint-related issues.

Potential Homeopathic Uses

If Hematite were to be used as a homeopathic remedy, its indications might include:

Psychological Symptoms: Anxiety, emotional stress, and lack of focus. It may also help in cases of emotional instability and lack of clarity.

Physical Symptoms: Blood health issues, detoxification needs, and immune system deficiencies.

Behavioral Symptoms: Difficulty in coping with stress, lack of motivation, and a tendency towards emotional imbalance.

Hematite's homeopathic profile would focus on its ability to ground, protect, and invigorate, making it suitable for addressing conditions related to stress, blood health, and overall well-being.

Conclusion

Hematite is a vital crystal in holistic healing, celebrated for its grounding beauty and versatile healing properties. Whether used for stress relief, mental clarity, or as a protective talisman, Hematite serves as a potent aid in achieving physical health and spiritual harmony. Like all alternative practices, these should be considered as complementary to conventional medical treatments.

Kämmererite: Comprehensive Guide on Spiritual and Physical Healing Properties

Overview

Kämmererite, known for its vibrant purple to pink hues, is a rare and captivating crystal valued for its high-frequency energy and spiritual properties. This gemstone is often associated with transformation and spiritual awakening. Kämmererite is celebrated for its ability to enhance intuition and promote overall well-being.

Spiritual and Psychic Benefits

Stress Relief and Calming: Kämmererite is renowned for its ability to alleviate stress and anxiety. Its high-frequency energy promotes a sense of peace and tranquility, helping to calm the mind and reduce emotional tension. This makes it an excellent companion for meditation and spiritual practices.

Intuition and Psychic Abilities: Connected to the third eye and crown chakras, Kämmererite enhances intuition and psychic abilities. It encourages deep spiritual insight and clarity, helping individuals to connect with their higher self and the universe.

Spiritual Transformation: Kämmererite is a stone of transformation and spiritual awakening. It supports the release of old patterns and the acceptance of new perspectives, facilitating profound changes in one's spiritual journey.

Enhancement of Healing Energies: Known for its ability to amplify healing energies, Kämmererite is used to enhance both personal energy and the effectiveness of other healing crystals. It is beneficial in promoting a balanced and harmonious energy flow during healing sessions.

Harmonization and Balance: Kämmererite aids in balancing the body's subtle energies. It aligns the chakras and stabilizes emotions, fostering a harmonious internal environment that supports spiritual and emotional well-being.

Versatile Use in Healing Practices: Utilized in various forms such as raw crystals, jewelry, and meditation tools, Kämmererite is a key component in holistic healing practices. It is often used in energy layouts to align and balance the body's energy centers.

Physical Healing Properties

Vitality and Energy: Kämmererite is believed to boost physical vitality and energy levels. It helps to invigorate the body, enhancing stamina and overall health.

Detoxification: Kämmererite aids in detoxifying the body, supporting liver function and cleansing the system of toxins. This contributes to improved metabolic health and overall well-being.

Immune System: Kämmererite is believed to enhance the immune system, helping the body to fight off illnesses more effectively. It supports the body's natural defenses and promotes overall health and vitality.

Cellular Regeneration: Kämmererite supports the body's natural healing processes by promoting cellular regeneration. It aids in the recovery from injuries and illnesses, speeding up the healing process.

Bone and Joint Health: Kämmererite supports bone and joint health, helping to strengthen bones and alleviate joint pain. It is beneficial for those dealing with arthritis and other joint-related issues .

Potential Homeopathic Uses

If Kämmererite were to be used as a homeopathic remedy, its indications might include:

Psychological Symptoms: Anxiety, emotional stress, and lack of clarity. It may also help in cases of emotional instability and spiritual confusion.

Physical Symptoms: Detoxification needs, immune system deficiencies, and joint pain.

Behavioral Symptoms: Difficulty in coping with stress, lack of motivation, and a tendency towards emotional imbalance.

Kämmererite's homeopathic profile would focus on its ability to transform, protect, and rejuvenate, making it suitable for addressing conditions related to stress, detoxification, and overall well-being.

Conclusion

Kämmererite is a vital crystal in holistic healing, celebrated for its vibrant beauty and versatile healing properties. Whether used for stress relief, spiritual transformation, or as an intuitive talisman, Kämmererite serves as a potent aid in achieving physical health and spiritual harmony. Like all alternative practices, these should be considered as complementary to conventional medical treatments.

Lodolite: Comprehensive Guide on Spiritual and Physical Healing Properties

Overview

Lodolite, also known as Garden Quartz or Shamanic Dream Quartz, is a unique crystal with inclusions that resemble miniature landscapes or gardens. This gemstone is often associated with healing and transformation. Lodolite is celebrated for its ability to enhance spiritual growth and promote overall well-being.

Spiritual and Psychic Benefits

Stress Relief and Calming: Lodolite is renowned for its ability to alleviate stress and anxiety. Its tranquil energy promotes a sense of peace and relaxation, helping to calm the mind and body. This makes it an excellent companion for meditation and spiritual practices.

Spiritual Growth: Connected to the crown and third eye chakras, Lodolite enhances spiritual growth and inner vision. It encourages deep introspection and clarity, helping individuals to connect with their higher self and the spiritual realm.

Transformation and Healing: Lodolite is a stone of transformation and healing. It supports the release of old patterns and facilitates the acceptance of new perspectives, aiding in profound personal and spiritual changes.

Enhancement of Healing Energies: Known for its ability to amplify healing energies, Lodolite is used to enhance both personal energy and the effectiveness of other healing crystals. It is beneficial in promoting a balanced and harmonious energy flow during healing sessions.

Harmonization and Balance: Lodolite aids in balancing the body's subtle energies. It aligns the chakras and stabilizes emotions, fostering a harmonious internal environment that supports emotional and spiritual well-being.

Versatile Use in Healing Practices: Utilized in various forms such as raw crystals, jewelry, and meditation tools, Lodolite is a key component

in holistic healing practices. It is often used in energy layouts to align and balance the body's energy centers.

Physical Healing Properties

Vitality and Energy: Lodolite is believed to boost physical vitality and energy levels. It helps to invigorate the body, enhancing stamina and overall health.

Detoxification: Lodolite aids in detoxifying the body, supporting liver function and cleansing the system of toxins. This contributes to improved metabolic health and overall well-being.

Immune System: Lodolite is believed to enhance the immune system, helping the body to fight off illnesses more effectively. It supports the body's natural defenses and promotes overall health and vitality.

Cellular Regeneration: Lodolite supports the body's natural healing processes by promoting cellular regeneration. It aids in the recovery from injuries and illnesses, speeding up the healing process.

Skin Health: Lodolite supports skin health by promoting cellular regeneration and healing. It aids in the treatment of skin conditions and improves the overall appearance of the skin.

Potential Homeopathic Uses

If Lodolite were to be used as a homeopathic remedy, its indications might include:

Psychological Symptoms: Anxiety, emotional stress, and lack of clarity. It may also help in cases of emotional instability and spiritual confusion.

Physical Symptoms: Detoxification needs, immune system deficiencies, and skin conditions.

Behavioral Symptoms: Difficulty in coping with stress, lack of motivation, and a tendency towards emotional imbalance.

Lodolite's homeopathic profile would focus on its ability to transform, protect, and rejuvenate, making it suitable for addressing conditions related to stress, detoxification, and overall well-being.

Conclusion

Lodolite is a vital crystal in holistic healing, celebrated for its unique beauty and versatile healing properties. Whether used for stress relief, spiritual growth, or as a transformative talisman, Lodolite serves as a potent aid in achieving physical health and spiritual harmony. Like all alternative practices, these should be considered as complementary to conventional medical treatments.

Psilomelane: Comprehensive Guide on Spiritual and Physical Healing Properties

Overview

Psilomelane, known for its striking black and silver banded appearance, is a powerful crystal valued for its grounding and protective energy. This gemstone is often associated with emotional healing and clarity. Psilomelane is celebrated for its ability to enhance mental focus and promote overall well-being.

Spiritual and Psychic Benefits

Stress Relief and Calming: Psilomelane is renowned for its ability to alleviate stress and anxiety. Its grounding energy promotes a sense of stability and calm, helping to clear the mind and reduce emotional tension. This makes it an excellent companion for meditation and stress management practices.

Emotional Healing: Connected to the root and sacral chakras, Psilomelane enhances emotional healing and resilience. It encourages the release of negative emotions and supports emotional balance, helping individuals to achieve a harmonious state of mind.

Mental Clarity: Psilomelane is a stone of mental clarity and focus. It supports clear thinking and decision-making, helping individuals to approach challenges with confidence and determination.

Enhancement of Healing Energies: Known for its ability to amplify healing energies, Psilomelane is used to enhance both personal energy and the effectiveness of other healing crystals. It is beneficial in promoting a balanced and harmonious energy flow during healing sessions.

Harmonization and Balance: Psilomelane aids in balancing the body's subtle energies. It aligns the chakras and stabilizes emotions, fostering a harmonious internal environment that supports emotional and physical well-being.

Versatile Use in Healing Practices: Utilized in various forms such as raw crystals, jewelry, and meditation tools, Psilomelane is a key component in holistic healing practices. It is often used in energy layouts to align and balance the body's energy centers.

Physical Healing Properties

Vitality and Energy: Psilomelane is believed to boost physical vitality and energy levels. It helps to invigorate the body, enhancing stamina and overall health.

Immune System: Psilomelane is believed to enhance the immune system, helping the body to fight off illnesses more effectively. It supports the body's natural defenses and promotes overall health and vitality.

Detoxification: Psilomelane aids in detoxifying the body, supporting liver function and cleansing the system of toxins. This contributes to improved metabolic health and overall well-being.

Bone and Joint Health: Psilomelane supports bone and joint health, helping to strengthen bones and alleviate joint pain. It is beneficial for those dealing with arthritis and other joint-related issues.

Healing and Regeneration: Psilomelane supports the body's natural healing processes by promoting cellular regeneration. It aids in the recovery from injuries and illnesses, speeding up the healing process.

Potential Homeopathic Uses

If Psilomelane were to be used as a homeopathic remedy, its indications might include:

Psychological Symptoms: Anxiety, emotional stress, and lack of clarity. It may also help in cases of emotional instability and difficulty focusing.

Physical Symptoms: Immune system deficiencies, detoxification needs, and joint pain.

Behavioral Symptoms: Difficulty in coping with stress, lack of motivation, and a tendency towards emotional imbalance.

Psilomelane's homeopathic profile would focus on its ability to ground, protect, and clarify, making it suitable for addressing conditions related to stress, immune health, and overall well-being.

Conclusion

Psilomelane is a vital crystal in holistic healing, celebrated for its grounding beauty and versatile healing properties. Whether used for stress relief, emotional healing, or as a protective talisman, Psilomelane serves as a potent aid in achieving physical health and spiritual harmony. Like all alternative practices, these should be considered as complementary to conventional medical treatments.

Realgar: Comprehensive Guide on Spiritual and Physical Healing Properties

Overview

Realgar, known for its vivid red to orange color, is a rare and powerful crystal valued for its transformative and energizing properties. This gemstone is often associated with passion and vitality. Realgar is celebrated for its ability to enhance creativity and promote overall well-being.

Spiritual and Psychic Benefits

Stress Relief and Calming: Realgar is renowned for its ability to alleviate stress and anxiety. Its vibrant energy promotes a sense of joy and enthusiasm, helping to uplift the spirit and dispel negative emotions. This makes it an excellent companion for meditation and stress management practices.

Creativity and Passion: Connected to the sacral chakra, Realgar enhances creativity and passion. It encourages self-expression and inspires new ideas, making it a powerful tool for artists and creators.

Transformation and Growth: Realgar is a stone of transformation and growth. It supports the release of old patterns and the acceptance of new perspectives, facilitating profound changes in one's personal and spiritual journey.

Enhancement of Healing Energies: Known for its ability to amplify healing energies, Realgar is used to enhance both personal energy and the effectiveness of other healing crystals. It is beneficial in promoting a balanced and harmonious energy flow during healing sessions.

Harmonization and Balance: Realgar aids in balancing the body's subtle energies. It aligns the chakras and stabilizes emotions, fostering a harmonious internal environment that supports emotional and physical well-being.

Versatile Use in Healing Practices: Utilized in various forms such as raw crystals, jewelry, and meditation tools, Realgar is a key component in holistic healing practices. It is often used in energy layouts to align and balance the body's energy centers.

Physical Healing Properties

Vitality and Energy: Realgar is believed to boost physical vitality and energy levels. It helps to invigorate the body, enhancing stamina and overall health.

Detoxification: Realgar aids in detoxifying the body, supporting liver function and cleansing the system of toxins. This contributes to improved metabolic health and overall well-being.

Immune System: Realgar is believed to enhance the immune system, helping the body to fight off illnesses more effectively. It supports the body's natural defenses and promotes overall health and vitality.

Reproductive Health: Realgar supports reproductive health, helping to balance hormonal levels and enhance fertility. It is beneficial for those dealing with reproductive issues.

Healing and Regeneration: Realgar supports the body's natural healing processes by promoting cellular regeneration. It aids in the recovery from injuries and illnesses, speeding up the healing process.

Potential Homeopathic Uses

If Realgar were to be used as a homeopathic remedy, its indications might include:

Psychological Symptoms: Anxiety, low self-esteem, and lack of motivation. It may also help in cases of emotional instability and lack of passion.

Physical Symptoms: Reproductive health issues, detoxification needs, and immune system deficiencies.

Behavioral Symptoms: Difficulty in coping with stress, lack of creativity, and a tendency towards emotional imbalance.

Realgar's homeopathic profile would focus on its ability to invigorate, transform, and inspire, making it suitable for addressing conditions related to stress, reproductive health, and overall well-being.

Conclusion

Realgar is a vital crystal in holistic healing, celebrated for its vibrant beauty and versatile healing properties. Whether used for stress relief, personal empowerment, or as a transformative talisman, Realgar serves as a potent aid in achieving physical health and spiritual harmony. Like all alternative practices, these should be considered as complementary to conventional medical treatments.

Wavellite: Comprehensive Guide on Spiritual and Physical Healing Properties

Overview

Wavellite, known for its beautiful radial clusters of green to yellow-green hues, is a unique crystal appreciated for its soothing and harmonizing energy. This gemstone is often associated with balance and insight. Wavellite is celebrated for its ability to enhance mental clarity and promote overall well-being.

Spiritual and Psychic Benefits

Stress Relief and Calming: Wavellite is renowned for its ability to alleviate stress and anxiety. Its calming energy promotes a sense of peace and relaxation, helping to clear the mind and reduce emotional tension. This makes it an excellent companion for meditation and stress management practices.

Mental Clarity: Connected to the heart and third eye chakras, Wavellite enhances mental clarity and insight. It encourages clear thinking and decision-making, helping individuals to approach challenges with confidence and understanding.

Emotional Balance: Wavellite is a stone of emotional balance and harmony. It supports the release of negative emotions and promotes emotional healing, helping individuals to achieve a harmonious state of mind.

Enhancement of Healing Energies: Known for its ability to amplify healing energies, Wavellite is used to enhance both personal energy and the effectiveness of other healing crystals. It is beneficial in promoting a balanced and harmonious energy flow during healing sessions.

Harmonization and Balance: Wavellite aids in balancing the body's subtle energies. It aligns the chakras and stabilizes emotions, fostering a harmonious internal environment that supports emotional and spiritual well-being.

Versatile Use in Healing Practices: Utilized in various forms such as raw crystals, jewelry, and meditation tools, Wavellite is a key component in holistic healing practices. It is often used in energy layouts to align and balance the body's energy centers.

Physical Healing Properties

Vitality and Energy: Wavellite is believed to boost physical vitality and energy levels. It helps to invigorate the body, enhancing stamina and overall health.

Immune System: Wavellite is believed to enhance the immune system, helping the body to fight off illnesses more effectively. It supports the body's natural defenses and promotes overall health and vitality.

Detoxification: Wavellite aids in detoxifying the body, supporting liver function and cleansing the system of toxins. This contributes to improved metabolic health and overall well-being.

Cellular Regeneration: Wavellite supports the body's natural healing processes by promoting cellular regeneration. It aids in the recovery from injuries and illnesses, speeding up the healing process.

Digestive Health: Wavellite supports digestive health by promoting a healthy digestive system. It helps to alleviate issues such as indigestion and stomach discomfort, contributing to overall digestive well-being.

Potential Homeopathic Uses

If Wavellite were to be used as a homeopathic remedy, its indications might include:

Psychological Symptoms: Anxiety, emotional stress, and lack of clarity. It may also help in cases of emotional instability and difficulty focusing.

Physical Symptoms: Immune system deficiencies, detoxification needs, and digestive issues.

Behavioral Symptoms: Difficulty in coping with stress, lack of motivation, and a tendency towards emotional imbalance.

Wavellite's homeopathic profile would focus on its ability to clarify, protect, and harmonize, making it suitable for addressing conditions related to stress, immune health, and overall well-being.

Conclusion

Wavellite is a vital crystal in holistic healing, celebrated for its soothing beauty and versatile healing properties. Whether used for stress relief, mental clarity, or as a harmonizing talisman, Wavellite serves as a potent aid in achieving physical health and spiritual harmony. Like all alternative practices, these should be considered as complementary to conventional medical treatments.

Bytownite: Comprehensive Guide on Spiritual and Physical Healing Properties

Overview

Bytownite, known for its translucent to opaque appearance with colors ranging from yellow to greenish-yellow, is a captivating crystal appreciated for its grounding and stabilizing energy. This gemstone is often associated with strength and clarity. Bytownite is celebrated for its ability to enhance mental focus and promote overall well-being.

Spiritual and Psychic Benefits

Stress Relief and Calming: Bytownite is renowned for its ability to alleviate stress and anxiety. Its grounding energy promotes a sense of stability and calm, helping to clear the mind and reduce emotional tension. This makes it an excellent companion for meditation and stress management practices.

Mental Clarity: Connected to the solar plexus and root chakras, Bytownite enhances mental clarity and focus. It encourages clear thinking and decision-making, helping individuals to approach challenges with confidence and determination.

Emotional Strength: Bytownite is a stone of emotional strength and resilience. It supports the release of negative emotions and promotes emotional balance, helping individuals to achieve a harmonious state of mind.

Enhancement of Healing Energies: Known for its ability to amplify healing energies, Bytownite is used to enhance both personal energy and the effectiveness of other healing crystals. It is beneficial

in promoting a balanced and harmonious energy flow during healing sessions.

Harmonization and Balance: Bytownite aids in balancing the body's subtle energies. It aligns the chakras and stabilizes emotions, fostering a harmonious internal environment that supports emotional and physical well-being.

Versatile Use in Healing Practices: Utilized in various forms such as raw crystals, jewelry, and meditation tools, Bytownite is a key component in holistic healing practices. It is often used in energy layouts to align and balance the body's energy centers.

Physical Healing Properties

Vitality and Energy: Bytownite is believed to boost physical vitality and energy levels. It helps to invigorate the body, enhancing stamina and overall health.

Digestive Health: Bytownite supports digestive health by promoting a healthy digestive system. It helps to alleviate issues such as indigestion and stomach discomfort, contributing to overall digestive well-being.

Detoxification: Bytownite aids in detoxifying the body, supporting liver function and cleansing the system of toxins. This contributes to improved metabolic health and overall well-being.

Immune System: Bytownite is believed to enhance the immune system, helping the body to fight off illnesses more effectively. It supports the body's natural defenses and promotes overall health and vitality.

Bone and Joint Health: Bytownite supports bone and joint health, helping to strengthen bones and alleviate joint pain. It is beneficial for those dealing with arthritis and other joint-related issues.

Potential Homeopathic Uses

If Bytownite were to be used as a homeopathic remedy, its indications might include:

Psychological Symptoms: Anxiety, emotional stress, and lack of clarity. It may also help in cases of emotional instability and difficulty focusing.

Physical Symptoms: Digestive health issues, detoxification needs, and immune system deficiencies.

Behavioral Symptoms: Difficulty in coping with stress, lack of motivation, and a tendency towards emotional imbalance.

Bytownite's homeopathic profile would focus on its ability to ground, protect, and harmonize, making it suitable for addressing conditions related to stress, digestive health, and overall well-being.

Conclusion

Bytownite is a vital crystal in holistic healing, celebrated for its grounding beauty and versatile healing properties. Whether used for stress relief, mental clarity, or as a strengthening talisman, Bytownite serves as a potent aid in achieving physical health and spiritual harmony. Like all alternative practices, these should be considered as complementary to conventional medical treatments.

Londonite: Comprehensive Guide on Spiritual and Physical Healing Properties

Overview

Londonite, known for its pale yellow to greenish hues and high luster, is a rare and exquisite crystal appreciated for its balancing and harmonizing energy. This gemstone is often associated with mental clarity and emotional balance. Londonite is celebrated for its ability to enhance focus and promote overall well-being.

Spiritual and Psychic Benefits

Stress Relief and Calming: Londonite is renowned for its ability to alleviate stress and anxiety. Its calming energy promotes a sense of peace and tranquility, helping to clear the mind and reduce emotional tension. This makes it an excellent companion for meditation and stress management practices.

Mental Clarity: Connected to the crown and third eye chakras, Londonite enhances mental clarity and focus. It encourages clear thinking and decision-making, helping individuals to approach challenges with confidence and determination.

Emotional Balance: Londonite is a stone of emotional balance and harmony. It supports the release of negative emotions and promotes emotional healing, helping individuals to achieve a harmonious state of mind.

Enhancement of Healing Energies: Known for its ability to amplify healing energies, Londonite is used to enhance both personal energy and the effectiveness of other healing crystals. It is beneficial in promoting a balanced and harmonious energy flow during healing sessions.

Harmonization and Balance: Londonite aids in balancing the body's subtle energies. It aligns the chakras and stabilizes emotions, fostering a harmonious internal environment that supports emotional and mental well-being.

Versatile Use in Healing Practices: Utilized in various forms such as raw crystals, jewelry, and meditation tools, Londonite is a key component in holistic healing practices. It is often used in energy layouts to align and balance the body's energy centers.

Physical Healing Properties

Vitality and Energy: Londonite is believed to boost physical vitality and energy levels. It helps to invigorate the body, enhancing stamina and overall health.

Detoxification: Londonite aids in detoxifying the body, supporting liver function and cleansing the system of toxins. This contributes to improved metabolic health and overall well-being.

Immune System: Londonite is believed to enhance the immune system, helping the body to fight off illnesses more effectively. It supports the body's natural defenses and promotes overall health and vitality.

Bone and Joint Health: Londonite supports bone and joint health, helping to strengthen bones and alleviate joint pain. It is beneficial for those dealing with arthritis and other joint-related issues.

Healing and Regeneration: Londonite supports the body's natural healing processes by promoting cellular regeneration. It aids in the recovery from injuries and illnesses, speeding up the healing process.

Potential Homeopathic Uses

If Londonite were to be used as a homeopathic remedy, its indications might include:

Psychological Symptoms: Anxiety, emotional stress, and lack of clarity. It may also help in cases of emotional instability and difficulty focusing.

Physical Symptoms: Detoxification needs, immune system deficiencies, and joint pain.

Behavioral Symptoms: Difficulty in coping with stress, lack of motivation, and a tendency towards emotional imbalance.

Londonite's homeopathic profile would focus on its ability to balance, protect, and clarify, making it suitable for addressing conditions related to stress, detoxification, and overall well-being.

Conclusion

Londonite is a vital crystal in holistic healing, celebrated for its exquisite beauty and versatile healing properties. Whether used for stress relief, mental clarity, or as a harmonizing talisman, Londonite serves as a potent aid in achieving physical health and spiritual harmony. Like all alternative practices, these should be considered as complementary to conventional medical treatments.

Muscovite: Comprehensive Guide on Spiritual and Physical Healing Properties

Overview

Muscovite, known for its silvery to pale yellow or greenish layers, is a captivating crystal appreciated for its reflective and protective energy. This gemstone is often associated with clarity and emotional balance. Muscovite is celebrated for its ability to enhance intuition and promote overall well-being.

Spiritual and Psychic Benefits

Stress Relief and Calming: Muscovite is renowned for its ability to alleviate stress and anxiety. Its reflective energy promotes a sense of peace and tranquility, helping to clear the mind and reduce emotional tension. This makes it an excellent companion for meditation and stress management practices.

Intuition and Spiritual Insight: Connected to the third eye and crown chakras, Muscovite enhances intuition and spiritual insight. It encourages clarity of thought and deep spiritual understanding, helping individuals to connect with their higher self and the spiritual realm.

Emotional Balance: Muscovite is a stone of emotional balance and harmony. It supports the release of negative emotions and promotes emotional healing, helping individuals to achieve a harmonious state of mind.

Enhancement of Healing Energies: Known for its ability to amplify healing energies, Muscovite is used to enhance both personal energy and the effectiveness of other healing crystals. It is beneficial in promoting a balanced and harmonious energy flow during healing sessions.

Harmonization and Balance: Muscovite aids in balancing the body's subtle energies. It aligns the chakras and stabilizes emotions, fostering a harmonious internal environment that supports emotional and spiritual well-being.

Versatile Use in Healing Practices: Utilized in various forms such as raw crystals, jewelry, and meditation tools, Muscovite is a key component in holistic healing practices. It is often used in energy layouts to align and balance the body's energy centers.

Physical Healing Properties

Vitality and Energy: Muscovite is believed to boost physical vitality and energy levels. It helps to invigorate the body, enhancing stamina and overall health.

Detoxification: Muscovite aids in detoxifying the body, supporting liver function and cleansing the system of toxins. This contributes to improved metabolic health and overall well-being.

Immune System: Muscovite is believed to enhance the immune system, helping the body to fight off illnesses more effectively. It supports the body's natural defenses and promotes overall health and vitality.

Skin Health: Muscovite supports skin health by promoting cellular regeneration and healing. It aids in the treatment of skin conditions and improves the overall appearance of the skin.

Healing and Regeneration: Muscovite supports the body's natural healing processes by promoting cellular regeneration. It aids in the recovery from injuries and illnesses, speeding up the healing process.

Potential Homeopathic Uses

If Muscovite were to be used as a homeopathic remedy, its indications might include:

Psychological Symptoms: Anxiety, emotional stress, and lack of clarity. It may also help in cases of emotional instability and difficulty focusing.

Physical Symptoms: Skin health issues, detoxification needs, and immune system deficiencies.

Behavioral Symptoms: Difficulty in coping with stress, lack of motivation, and a tendency towards emotional imbalance.

Muscovite's homeopathic profile would focus on its ability to clarify, protect, and heal, making it suitable for addressing conditions related to stress, skin health, and overall well-being.

Conclusion

Muscovite is a vital crystal in holistic healing, celebrated for its reflective beauty and versatile healing properties. Whether used for stress relief, intuition enhancement, or as a protective talisman, Muscovite serves as a potent aid in achieving physical health and spiritual harmony. Like all alternative practices, these should be considered as complementary to conventional medical treatments.

Petalite: Comprehensive Guide on Spiritual and Physical Healing Properties

Overview

Petalite, known for its clear to milky white or pinkish hues, is a serene and high-vibrational crystal valued for its calming and protective energy. This gemstone is often associated with spiritual awakening and peace. Petalite is celebrated for its ability to enhance meditation and promote overall well-being.

Spiritual and Psychic Benefits

Stress Relief and Calming: Petalite is renowned for its ability to alleviate stress and anxiety. Its calming energy promotes a sense of peace and tranquility, helping to clear the mind and reduce emotional tension. This makes it an excellent companion for meditation and spiritual practices.

Spiritual Awakening: Connected to the crown and third eye chakras, Petalite enhances spiritual awakening and higher consciousness. It encourages deep spiritual insight and clarity, helping individuals to connect with their higher self and the spiritual realm.

Protection: Petalite is a stone of protection, especially during spiritual work. It helps to create a protective shield around the aura, safeguarding against negative energies and psychic attacks.

Enhancement of Healing Energies: Known for its ability to amplify healing energies, Petalite is used to enhance both personal energy and the effectiveness of other healing crystals. It is beneficial in promoting a balanced and harmonious energy flow during healing sessions.

Harmonization and Balance: Petalite aids in balancing the body's subtle energies. It aligns the chakras and stabilizes emotions, fostering a harmonious internal environment that supports emotional and spiritual well-being.

Versatile Use in Healing Practices: Utilized in various forms such as raw crystals, jewelry, and meditation tools, Petalite is a key component

in holistic healing practices. It is often used in energy layouts to align and balance the body's energy centers.

Physical Healing Properties

Vitality and Energy: Petalite is believed to boost physical vitality and energy levels. It helps to invigorate the body, enhancing stamina and overall health.

Nervous System: Petalite supports the nervous system, helping to alleviate issues such as anxiety and stress-related disorders. It promotes a calm and balanced state of mind.

Detoxification: Petalite aids in detoxifying the body, supporting liver function and cleansing the system of toxins. This contributes to improved metabolic health and overall well-being.

Immune System: Petalite is believed to enhance the immune system, helping the body to fight off illnesses more effectively. It supports the body's natural defenses and promotes overall health and vitality.

Healing and Regeneration: Petalite supports the body's natural healing processes by promoting cellular regeneration. It aids in the recovery from injuries and illnesses, speeding up the healing process.

Potential Homeopathic Uses

If Petalite were to be used as a homeopathic remedy, its indications might include:

Psychological Symptoms: Anxiety, emotional stress, and lack of clarity. It may also help in cases of emotional instability and spiritual confusion.

Physical Symptoms: Nervous system issues, detoxification needs, and immune system deficiencies.

Behavioral Symptoms: Difficulty in coping with stress, lack of motivation, and a tendency towards emotional imbalance.

Petalite's homeopathic profile would focus on its ability to soothe, protect, and rejuvenate, making it suitable for addressing conditions related to stress, nervous system health, and overall well-being.

Conclusion

Petalite is a vital crystal in holistic healing, celebrated for its serene beauty and versatile healing properties. Whether used for stress relief, spiritual awakening, or as a protective talisman, Petalite serves as a potent aid in achieving physical health and spiritual harmony. Like all alternative practices, these should be considered as complementary to conventional medical treatments.

Roselite: Comprehensive Guide on Spiritual and Physical Healing Properties

Overview

Roselite, known for its vibrant pink to reddish hues, is a rare and enchanting crystal valued for its loving and nurturing energy. This gemstone is often associated with emotional healing and compassion. Roselite is celebrated for its ability to enhance love and promote overall well-being.

Spiritual and Psychic Benefits

Stress Relief and Calming: Roselite is renowned for its ability to alleviate stress and anxiety. Its loving energy promotes a sense of peace and comfort, helping to clear the mind and reduce emotional tension. This makes it an excellent companion for meditation and emotional healing practices.

Emotional Healing: Connected to the heart chakra, Roselite enhances emotional healing and compassion. It encourages the release of negative emotions and supports emotional balance, helping individuals to achieve a harmonious state of mind.

Love and Compassion: Roselite is a stone of love and compassion. It supports the development of loving relationships and encourages empathy and understanding. It is beneficial for enhancing self-love and acceptance.

Enhancement of Healing Energies: Known for its ability to amplify healing energies, Roselite is used to enhance both personal energy and the effectiveness of other healing crystals. It is beneficial

in promoting a balanced and harmonious energy flow during healing sessions.

Harmonization and Balance: Roselite aids in balancing the body's subtle energies. It aligns the chakras and stabilizes emotions, fostering a harmonious internal environment that supports emotional and spiritual well-being.

Versatile Use in Healing Practices: Utilized in various forms such as raw crystals, jewelry, and meditation tools, Roselite is a key component in holistic healing practices. It is often used in energy layouts to align and balance the body's energy centers.

Physical Healing Properties

Vitality and Energy: Roselite is believed to boost physical vitality and energy levels. It helps to invigorate the body, enhancing stamina and overall health.

Heart Health: This crystal supports heart health by promoting a healthy cardiovascular system. It helps to alleviate issues such as heartache and emotional stress, contributing to overall heart health.

Detoxification: Roselite aids in detoxifying the body, supporting liver function and cleansing the system of toxins. This contributes to improved metabolic health and overall well-being.

Immune System: Roselite is believed to enhance the immune system, helping the body to fight off illnesses more effectively. It supports the body's natural defenses and promotes overall health and vitality.

Healing and Regeneration: Roselite supports the body's natural healing processes by promoting cellular regeneration. It aids in the recovery from injuries and illnesses, speeding up the healing process.

Potential Homeopathic Uses

If Roselite were to be used as a homeopathic remedy, its indications might include:

Psychological Symptoms: Anxiety, emotional stress, and lack of self-love. It may also help in cases of emotional instability and difficulty in relationships.

Physical Symptoms: Heart health issues, detoxification needs, and immune system deficiencies.

Behavioral Symptoms: Difficulty in coping with stress, lack of empathy, and a tendency towards emotional imbalance.

Roselite's homeopathic profile would focus on its ability to heal, protect, and nurture, making it suitable for addressing conditions related to stress, heart health, and overall well-being.

Conclusion

Roselite is a vital crystal in holistic healing, celebrated for its vibrant beauty and versatile healing properties. Whether used for stress relief, emotional healing, or as a loving talisman, Roselite serves as a potent aid in achieving physical health and spiritual harmony. Like all alternative practices, these should be considered as complementary to conventional medical treatments.

Siderite: Comprehensive Guide on Spiritual and Physical Healing Properties

Overview

Siderite, known for its earthy brown to yellowish hues, is a grounding and stabilizing crystal valued for its protective and nurturing energy. This gemstone is often associated with strength and resilience. Siderite is celebrated for its ability to enhance focus and promote overall well-being.

Spiritual and Psychic Benefits

Stress Relief and Calming: Siderite is renowned for its ability to alleviate stress and anxiety. Its grounding energy promotes a sense of stability and calm, helping to clear the mind and reduce emotional tension. This makes it an excellent companion for meditation and stress management practices.

Grounding and Protection: Connected to the root chakra, Siderite enhances grounding and protection. It encourages a strong connection to the earth, helping individuals to feel secure and centered.

Mental Clarity: Siderite is a stone of mental clarity and focus. It supports clear thinking and decision-making, helping individuals to approach challenges with confidence and determination.

Enhancement of Healing Energies: Known for its ability to amplify healing energies, Siderite is used to enhance both personal energy and the effectiveness of other healing crystals. It is beneficial in promoting a balanced and harmonious energy flow during healing sessions.

Harmonization and Balance: Siderite aids in balancing the body's subtle energies. It aligns the chakras and stabilizes emotions, fostering a harmonious internal environment that supports emotional and physical well-being.

Versatile Use in Healing Practices: Utilized in various forms such as raw crystals, jewelry, and meditation tools, Siderite is a key component in holistic healing practices. It is often used in energy layouts to align and balance the body's energy centers.

Physical Healing Properties

Vitality and Energy: Siderite is believed to boost physical vitality and energy levels. It helps to invigorate the body, enhancing stamina and overall health.

Bone and Joint Health: Siderite supports bone and joint health, helping to strengthen bones and alleviate joint pain. It is beneficial for those dealing with arthritis and other joint-related issues.

Detoxification: Siderite aids in detoxifying the body, supporting liver function and cleansing the system of toxins. This contributes to improved metabolic health and overall well-being.

Immune System: Siderite is believed to enhance the immune system, helping the body to fight off illnesses more effectively. It

supports the body's natural defenses and promotes overall health and vitality.

Cellular Regeneration: Siderite supports the body's natural healing processes by promoting cellular regeneration. It aids in the recovery from injuries and illnesses, speeding up the healing process.

Potential Homeopathic Uses

If Siderite were to be used as a homeopathic remedy, its indications might include:

Psychological Symptoms: Anxiety, emotional stress, and lack of clarity. It may also help in cases of emotional instability and difficulty focusing.

Physical Symptoms: Bone and joint health issues, detoxification needs, and immune system deficiencies.

Behavioral Symptoms: Difficulty in coping with stress, lack of motivation, and a tendency towards emotional imbalance.

Siderite's homeopathic profile would focus on its ability to ground, protect, and clarify, making it suitable for addressing conditions related to stress, bone health, and overall well-being.

Conclusion

Siderite is a vital crystal in holistic healing, celebrated for its grounding beauty and versatile healing properties. Whether used for stress relief, mental clarity, or as a protective talisman, Siderite serves as a potent aid in achieving physical health and spiritual harmony. Like all alternative practices, these should be considered as complementary to conventional medical treatments.

Tantalite: Comprehensive Guide on Spiritual and Physical Healing Properties

Overview

Tantalite, known for its dark to black metallic appearance, is a powerful and grounding crystal valued for its protective and stabilizing energy. This gemstone is often associated with strength and resilience.

Tantalite is celebrated for its ability to enhance focus and promote overall well-being.

Spiritual and Psychic Benefits

Stress Relief and Calming: Tantalite is renowned for its ability to alleviate stress and anxiety. Its grounding energy promotes a sense of stability and calm, helping to clear the mind and reduce emotional tension. This makes it an excellent companion for meditation and stress management practices.

Grounding and Protection: Connected to the root chakra, Tantalite enhances grounding and protection. It encourages a strong connection to the earth, helping individuals to feel secure and centered.

Mental Clarity: Tantalite is a stone of mental clarity and focus. It supports clear thinking and decision-making, helping individuals to approach challenges with confidence and determination.

Enhancement of Healing Energies: Known for its ability to amplify healing energies, Tantalite is used to enhance both personal energy and the effectiveness of other healing crystals. It is beneficial in promoting a balanced and harmonious energy flow during healing sessions.

Harmonization and Balance: Tantalite aids in balancing the body's subtle energies. It aligns the chakras and stabilizes emotions, fostering a harmonious internal environment that supports emotional and physical well-being.

Versatile Use in Healing Practices: Utilized in various forms such as raw crystals, jewelry, and meditation tools, Tantalite is a key component in holistic healing practices. It is often used in energy layouts to align and balance the body's energy centers.

Physical Healing Properties

Vitality and Energy: Tantalite is believed to boost physical vitality and energy levels. It helps to invigorate the body, enhancing stamina and overall health.

Bone and Joint Health: Tantalite supports bone and joint health, helping to strengthen bones and alleviate joint pain. It is beneficial for those dealing with arthritis and other joint-related issues.

Detoxification: Tantalite aids in detoxifying the body, supporting liver function and cleansing the system of toxins. This contributes to improved metabolic health and overall well-being.

Immune System: Tantalite is believed to enhance the immune system, helping the body to fight off illnesses more effectively.

It supports the body's natural defenses and promotes overall health and vitality.

Cellular Regeneration: Tantalite supports the body's natural healing processes by promoting cellular regeneration. It aids in the recovery from injuries and illnesses, speeding up the healing process.

Potential Homeopathic Uses

If Tantalite were to be used as a homeopathic remedy, its indications might include:

Psychological Symptoms: Anxiety, emotional stress, and lack of clarity. It may also help in cases of emotional instability and difficulty focusing.

Physical Symptoms: Bone and joint health issues, detoxification needs, and immune system deficiencies.

Behavioral Symptoms: Difficulty in coping with stress, lack of motivation, and a tendency towards emotional imbalance.

Tantalite's homeopathic profile would focus on its ability to ground, protect, and clarify, making it suitable for addressing conditions related to stress, bone health, and overall well-being.

Conclusion

Tantalite is a vital crystal in holistic healing, celebrated for its grounding beauty and versatile healing properties. Whether used for stress relief, mental clarity, or as a protective talisman, Tantalite serves as a potent aid in achieving physical health and spiritual harmony. Like all alternative practices, these should be considered as complementary to conventional medical treatments.

Heliodor: Comprehensive Guide on Spiritual and Physical Healing Properties

Overview

Heliodor, known for its brilliant yellow to golden hues, is a vibrant crystal valued for its energizing and uplifting energy. This gemstone is often associated with clarity and personal power. Heliodor is celebrated for its ability to enhance confidence and promote overall well-being.

Spiritual and Psychic Benefits

Stress Relief and Calming: Heliodor is renowned for its ability to alleviate stress and anxiety. Its uplifting energy promotes a sense of joy and optimism, helping to clear the mind and reduce emotional tension. This makes it an excellent companion for meditation and stress management practices.

Personal Power and Confidence: Connected to the solar plexus chakra, Heliodor enhances personal power and confidence. It encourages self-expression and assertiveness, helping individuals to pursue their goals with determination and enthusiasm.

Clarity and Insight: Heliodor is a stone of clarity and insight. It supports clear thinking and decision-making, helping individuals to approach challenges with confidence and understanding.

Enhancement of Healing Energies: Known for its ability to amplify healing energies, Heliodor is used to enhance both personal energy and the effectiveness of other healing crystals. It is beneficial in promoting a balanced and harmonious energy flow during healing sessions.

Harmonization and Balance: Heliodor aids in balancing the body's subtle energies. It aligns the chakras and stabilizes emotions, fostering a harmonious internal environment that supports emotional and mental well-being.

Versatile Use in Healing Practices: Utilized in various forms such as raw crystals, jewelry, and meditation tools, Heliodor is a key component in holistic healing practices. It is often used in energy layouts to align and balance the body's energy centers.

Physical Healing Properties

Vitality and Energy: Heliodor is believed to boost physical vitality and energy levels. It helps to invigorate the body, enhancing stamina and overall health.

Digestive Health: Heliodor supports digestive health by promoting a healthy digestive system. It helps to alleviate issues such as indigestion and stomach discomfort, contributing to overall digestive well-being.

Immune System: Heliodor is believed to enhance the immune system, helping the body to fight off illnesses more effectively. It supports the body's natural defenses and promotes overall health and vitality.

Detoxification: Heliodor aids in detoxifying the body, supporting liver function and cleansing the system of toxins. This contributes to improved metabolic health and overall well-being.

Healing and Regeneration: Heliodor supports the body's natural healing processes by promoting cellular regeneration. It aids in the recovery from injuries and illnesses, speeding up the healing process.

Potential Homeopathic Uses

If Heliodor were to be used as a homeopathic remedy, its indications might include:

Psychological Symptoms: Anxiety, low self-esteem, and lack of motivation. It may also help in cases of emotional instability and lack of clarity.

Physical Symptoms: Digestive health issues, immune system deficiencies, and detoxification needs.

Behavioral Symptoms: Difficulty in coping with stress, lack of confidence, and a tendency towards emotional imbalance.

Heliodor's homeopathic profile would focus on its ability to invigorate, protect, and clarify, making it suitable for addressing conditions related to stress, digestive health, and overall well-being.

Conclusion

Heliodor is a vital crystal in holistic healing, celebrated for its vibrant beauty and versatile healing properties. Whether used for stress relief, personal empowerment, or as a clarifying talisman, Heliodor serves as a potent aid in achieving physical health and spiritual harmony. Like all alternative practices, these should be considered as complementary to conventional medical treatments.

Andalusite: Comprehensive Guide on Spiritual and Physical Healing Properties

Overview

Andalusite, known for its pleochroic properties that display different colors when viewed from different angles, is a unique and captivating crystal valued for its balancing and protective energy. This gemstone is often associated with clarity and transformation. Andalusite is celebrated for its ability to enhance focus and promote overall well-being.

Spiritual and Psychic Benefits

Stress Relief and Calming: Andalusite is renowned for its ability to alleviate stress and anxiety. Its grounding energy promotes a sense of stability and calm, helping to clear the mind and reduce emotional tension. This makes it an excellent companion for meditation and stress management practices.

Mental Clarity and Focus: Connected to the root and solar plexus chakras, Andalusite enhances mental clarity and focus. It encourages clear thinking and decision-making, helping individuals to approach challenges with confidence and determination.

Transformation and Balance: Andalusite is a stone of transformation and balance. It supports the release of old patterns and facilitates the acceptance of new perspectives, aiding in profound personal and spiritual changes.

Enhancement of Healing Energies: Known for its ability to amplify healing energies, Andalusite is used to enhance both personal energy and the effectiveness of other healing crystals. It is beneficial in promoting a balanced and harmonious energy flow during healing sessions.

Harmonization and Balance: Andalusite aids in balancing the body's subtle energies. It aligns the chakras and stabilizes emotions, fostering a harmonious internal environment that supports emotional and mental well-being.

Versatile Use in Healing Practices: Utilized in various forms such as raw crystals, jewelry, and meditation tools, Andalusite is a key component in holistic healing practices. It is often used in energy layouts to align and balance the body's energy centers.

Physical Healing Properties

Vitality and Energy: Andalusite is believed to boost physical vitality and energy levels. It helps to invigorate the body, enhancing stamina and overall health.

Detoxification: Andalusite aids in detoxifying the body, supporting liver function and cleansing the system of toxins. This contributes to improved metabolic health and overall well-being.

Immune System: Andalusite is believed to enhance the immune system, helping the body to fight off illnesses more effectively. It supports the body's natural defenses and promotes overall health and vitality.

Bone and Joint Health: Andalusite supports bone and joint health, helping to strengthen bones and alleviate joint pain. It is beneficial for those dealing with arthritis and other joint-related issues.

Healing and Regeneration: Andalusite supports the body's natural healing processes by promoting cellular regeneration. It aids in the recovery from injuries and illnesses, speeding up the healing process.

Potential Homeopathic Uses

If Andalusite were to be used as a homeopathic remedy, its indications might include:

Psychological Symptoms: Anxiety, emotional stress, and lack of clarity. It may also help in cases of emotional instability and difficulty focusing.

Physical Symptoms: Detoxification needs, immune system deficiencies, and joint pain.

Behavioral Symptoms: Difficulty in coping with stress, lack of motivation, and a tendency towards emotional imbalance.

Andalusite's homeopathic profile would focus on its ability to transform, protect, and clarify, making it suitable for addressing conditions related to stress, detoxification, and overall well-being.

Conclusion

Andalusite is a vital crystal in holistic healing, celebrated for its unique beauty and versatile healing properties. Whether used for stress relief, mental clarity, or as a transformative talisman, Andalusite serves as a potent aid in achieving physical health and spiritual harmony. Like all alternative practices, these should be considered as complementary to conventional medical treatments.

Larvikite: Comprehensive Guide on Spiritual and Physical Healing Properties

Overview

Larvikite, known for its stunning blue and silver flashes within a dark matrix, is a grounding crystal valued for its protective and stabilizing energy. This gemstone is often associated with mental clarity and spiritual growth. Larvikite is celebrated for its ability to enhance psychic abilities and promote overall well-being.

Spiritual and Psychic Benefits

Stress Relief and Calming: Larvikite is renowned for its ability to alleviate stress and anxiety. Its grounding energy promotes a sense of stability and calm, helping to clear the mind and reduce emotional tension. This makes it an excellent companion for meditation and stress management practices.

Psychic Abilities: Connected to the third eye and crown chakras, Larvikite enhances psychic abilities and intuition. It encourages deep spiritual insight and clarity, helping individuals to connect with their higher self and the spiritual realm.

Spiritual Growth: Larvikite is a stone of spiritual growth and transformation. It supports the release of old patterns and the acceptance of new perspectives, facilitating profound changes in one's spiritual journey.

Enhancement of Healing Energies: Known for its ability to amplify healing energies, Larvikite is used to enhance both personal energy and the effectiveness of other healing crystals. It is beneficial in promoting a balanced and harmonious energy flow during healing sessions.

Harmonization and Balance: Larvikite aids in balancing the body's subtle energies. It aligns the chakras and stabilizes emotions, fostering a harmonious internal environment that supports emotional and spiritual well-being.

Versatile Use in Healing Practices: Utilized in various forms such as raw crystals, jewelry, and meditation tools, Larvikite is a key component in holistic healing practices. It is often used in energy layouts to align and balance the body's energy centers.

Physical Healing Properties

Vitality and Energy: Larvikite is believed to boost physical vitality and energy levels. It helps to invigorate the body, enhancing stamina and overall health.

Detoxification: Larvikite aids in detoxifying the body, supporting liver function and cleansing the system of toxins. This contributes to improved metabolic health and overall well-being.

Immune System: Larvikite is believed to enhance the immune system, helping the body to fight off illnesses more effectively. It supports the body's natural defenses and promotes overall health and vitality.

Skin Health: Larvikite supports skin health by promoting cellular regeneration and healing. It aids in the treatment of skin conditions and improves the overall appearance of the skin.

Healing and Regeneration: Larvikite supports the body's natural healing processes by promoting cellular regeneration. It aids in the recovery from injuries and illnesses, speeding up the healing process.

Potential Homeopathic Uses

If Larvikite were to be used as a homeopathic remedy, its indications might include:

Psychological Symptoms: Anxiety, emotional stress, and lack of clarity. It may also help in cases of emotional instability and spiritual confusion.

Physical Symptoms: Detoxification needs, immune system deficiencies, and skin conditions.

Behavioral Symptoms: Difficulty in coping with stress, lack of motivation, and a tendency towards emotional imbalance.

Larvikite's homeopathic profile would focus on its ability to ground, protect, and rejuvenate, making it suitable for addressing conditions related to stress, detoxification, and overall well-being.

Conclusion

Larvikite is a vital crystal in holistic healing, celebrated for its stunning beauty and versatile healing properties. Whether used for stress relief, psychic enhancement, or as a protective talisman, Larvikite serves as a potent aid in achieving physical health and spiritual harmony. Like all alternative practices, these should be considered as complementary to conventional medical treatments.

Chalcopyrite: Comprehensive Guide on Spiritual and Physical Healing Properties

Overview

Chalcopyrite, known for its vibrant metallic hues of gold, green, and blue, is a powerful crystal valued for its transformative and energizing energy. This gemstone is often associated with abundance and spiritual growth. Chalcopyrite is celebrated for its ability to enhance creativity and promote overall well-being.

Spiritual and Psychic Benefits

Stress Relief and Calming: Chalcopyrite is renowned for its ability to alleviate stress and anxiety. Its vibrant energy promotes a sense of joy and enthusiasm, helping to uplift the spirit and dispel negative emotions. This makes it an excellent companion for meditation and stress management practices.

Creativity and Abundance: Connected to the solar plexus and crown chakras, Chalcopyrite enhances creativity and attracts abundance. It encourages self-expression and inspires new ideas, making it a powerful tool for artists and creators.

Spiritual Growth: Chalcopyrite is a stone of spiritual growth and transformation. It supports the release of old patterns and the acceptance of new perspectives, facilitating profound changes in one's spiritual journey.

Enhancement of Healing Energies: Known for its ability to amplify healing energies, Chalcopyrite is used to enhance both personal energy and the effectiveness of other healing crystals. It is beneficial in promoting a balanced and harmonious energy flow during healing sessions.

Harmonization and Balance: Chalcopyrite aids in balancing the body's subtle energies. It aligns the chakras and stabilizes emotions, fostering a harmonious internal environment that supports emotional and spiritual well-being.

Versatile Use in Healing Practices: Utilized in various forms such as raw crystals, jewelry, and meditation tools, Chalcopyrite is a key component in holistic healing practices. It is often used in energy layouts to align and balance the body's energy centers.

Physical Healing Properties

Vitality and Energy: Chalcopyrite is believed to boost physical vitality and energy levels. It helps to invigorate the body, enhancing stamina and overall health.

Detoxification: Chalcopyrite aids in detoxifying the body, supporting liver function and cleansing the system of toxins. This contributes to improved metabolic health and overall well-being.

Immune System: Chalcopyrite is believed to enhance the immune system, helping the body to fight off illnesses more effectively. It supports the body's natural defenses and promotes overall health and vitality.

Cellular Regeneration: Chalcopyrite supports the body's natural healing processes by promoting cellular regeneration. It aids in the recovery from injuries and illnesses, speeding up the healing process.

Nervous System: Chalcopyrite supports the nervous system, helping to alleviate issues such as anxiety and stress-related disorders. It promotes a calm and balanced state of mind.

Potential Homeopathic Uses

If Chalcopyrite were to be used as a homeopathic remedy, its indications might include:

Psychological Symptoms : Anxiety, low self-esteem, and lack of motivation. It may also help in cases of emotional instability and lack of clarity.

Physical Symptoms: Detoxification needs, immune system deficiencies, and nervous system issues.

Behavioral Symptoms: Difficulty in coping with stress, lack of creativity, and a tendency towards emotional imbalance.

Chalcopyrite's homeopathic profile would focus on its ability to invigorate, protect, and transform, making it suitable for addressing conditions related to stress, detoxification, and overall well-being.

Conclusion

Chalcopyrite is a vital crystal in holistic healing, celebrated for its vibrant beauty and versatile healing properties. Whether used for stress relief, personal empowerment, or as a transformative talisman, Chalcopyrite serves as a potent aid in achieving physical health and spiritual harmony. Like all alternative practices, these should be considered as complementary to conventional medical treatments.

Diopside: Comprehensive Guide on Spiritual and Physical Healing Properties

Overview

Diopside, known for its rich green color and vitreous luster, is a captivating crystal valued for its healing and restorative energy. This gemstone is often associated with emotional healing and balance. Diopside is celebrated for its ability to enhance compassion and promote overall well-being.

Spiritual and Psychic Benefits

Stress Relief and Calming: Diopside is renowned for its ability to alleviate stress and anxiety. Its soothing energy promotes a sense of peace and tranquility, helping to calm the mind and body. This makes it an excellent companion for meditation and emotional healing practices.

Emotional Healing: Connected to the heart chakra, Diopside enhances emotional healing and compassion. It encourages the release of negative emotions and supports emotional balance, helping individuals to achieve a harmonious state of mind.

Compassion and Empathy: Diopside is a stone of compassion and empathy. It supports the development of loving relationships and encourages understanding and acceptance. It is beneficial for enhancing self-love and nurturing.

Enhancement of Healing Energies: Known for its ability to amplify healing energies, Diopside is used to enhance both personal energy and the effectiveness of other healing crystals. It is beneficial in promoting a balanced and harmonious energy flow during healing sessions.

Harmonization and Balance: Diopside aids in balancing the body's subtle energies. It aligns the chakras and stabilizes emotions, fostering a harmonious internal environment that supports emotional and spiritual well-being.

Versatile Use in Healing Practices: Utilized in various forms such as raw crystals, jewelry, and meditation tools, Diopside is a key component in holistic healing practices. It is often used in energy layouts to align and balance the body's energy centers.

Physical Healing Properties

Vitality and Energy: Diopside is believed to boost physical vitality and energy levels. It helps to invigorate the body, enhancing stamina and overall health.

Bone and Muscle Health: Diopside supports bone and muscle health, helping to strengthen bones and alleviate muscle pain. It is beneficial for those dealing with fractures and muscle-related issues.

Detoxification: Diopside aids in detoxifying the body, supporting liver function and cleansing the system of toxins. This contributes to improved metabolic health and overall well-being.

Immune System: Diopside is believed to enhance the immune system, helping the body to fight off illnesses more effectively. It supports the body's natural defenses and promotes overall health and vitality.

Healing and Regeneration: Diopside supports the body's natural healing processes by promoting cellular regeneration. It aids in the recovery from injuries and illnesses, speeding up the healing process.

Potential Homeopathic Uses

If Diopside were to be used as a homeopathic remedy, its indications might include:

Psychological Symptoms: Anxiety, emotional stress, and lack of compassion. It may also help in cases of emotional instability and difficulty in relationships.

Physical Symptoms: Bone and muscle health issues, detoxification needs, and immune system deficiencies.

Behavioral Symptoms: Difficulty in coping with stress, lack of empathy, and a tendency towards emotional imbalance.

Diopside's homeopathic profile would focus on its ability to heal, protect, and nurture, making it suitable for addressing conditions related to stress, bone health, and overall well-being.

Conclusion

Diopside is a vital crystal in holistic healing, celebrated for its rich beauty and versatile healing properties. Whether used for stress relief, emotional healing, or as a compassionate talisman, Diopside serves as a potent aid in achieving physical health and spiritual harmony. Like all alternative practices, these should be considered as complementary to conventional medical treatments.

Ekanite: Comprehensive Guide on Spiritual and Physical Healing Properties

Overview

Ekanite, known for its green to yellow-green hues and sometimes slightly radioactive properties, is a rare and intriguing crystal valued for its transformative and stabilizing energy. This gemstone is often associated with spiritual growth and clarity. Ekanite is celebrated for its ability to enhance intuition and promote overall well-being.

Spiritual and Psychic Benefits

Stress Relief and Calming: Ekanite is renowned for its ability to alleviate stress and anxiety. Its stabilizing energy promotes a sense of calm and balance, helping to clear the mind and reduce emotional tension. This makes it an excellent companion for meditation and stress management practices.

Intuition and Spiritual Growth: Connected to the third eye and crown chakras, Ekanite enhances intuition and spiritual growth. It encourages deep spiritual insight and clarity, helping individuals to connect with their higher self and the universe.

Transformation and Clarity: Ekanite is a stone of transformation and clarity. It supports the release of old patterns and facilitates the acceptance of new perspectives, aiding in profound personal and spiritual changes.

Enhancement of Healing Energies: Known for its ability to amplify healing energies, Ekanite is used to enhance both personal energy and the effectiveness of other healing crystals. It is beneficial in promoting a balanced and harmonious energy flow during healing sessions.

Harmonization and Balance: Ekanite aids in balancing the body's subtle energies. It aligns the chakras and stabilizes emotions, fostering a harmonious internal environment that supports emotional and spiritual well-being.

Versatile Use in Healing Practices: Utilized in various forms such as raw crystals, jewelry, and meditation tools, Ekanite is a key component in holistic healing practices. It is often used in energy layouts to align and balance the body's energy centers.

Physical Healing Properties

Vitality and Energy: Ekanite is believed to boost physical vitality and energy levels. It helps to invigorate the body, enhancing stamina and overall health.

Detoxification: Ekanite aids in detoxifying the body, supporting liver function and cleansing the system of toxins. This contributes to improved metabolic health and overall well-being.

Immune System: Ekanite is believed to enhance the immune system, helping the body to fight off illnesses more effectively. It supports the body's natural defenses and promotes overall health and vitality.

Bone and Joint Health: Ekanite supports bone and joint health, helping to strengthen bones and alleviate joint pain. It is beneficial for those dealing with arthritis and other joint-related issues.

Cellular Regeneration: Ekanite supports the body's natural healing processes by promoting cellular regeneration. It aids in the recovery from injuries and illnesses, speeding up the healing process.

Potential Homeopathic Uses

If Ekanite were to be used as a homeopathic remedy, its indications might include:

Psychological Symptoms: Anxiety, emotional stress, and lack of clarity. It may also help in cases of emotional instability and spiritual confusion.

Physical Symptoms: Detoxification needs, immune system deficiencies, and joint pain.

Behavioral Symptoms: Difficulty in coping with stress, lack of motivation, and a tendency towards emotional imbalance.

Ekanite's homeopathic profile would focus on its ability to transform, protect, and rejuvenate, making it suitable for addressing conditions related to stress, detoxification, and overall well-being.

Conclusion

Ekanite is a vital crystal in holistic healing, celebrated for its transformative beauty and versatile healing properties. Whether used for stress relief, spiritual growth, or as a clarifying talisman, Ekanite serves as a potent aid in achieving physical health and spiritual harmony. Like all alternative practices, these should be considered as complementary to conventional medical treatments.

Marcasite: Comprehensive Guide on Spiritual and Physical Healing Properties

Overview

Marcasite, known for its metallic luster and pale brass-yellow color, is a fascinating crystal appreciated for its grounding and protective energy. This gemstone is often associated with clarity and willpower. Marcasite is celebrated for its ability to enhance mental focus and promote overall well-being.

Spiritual and Psychic Benefits

Stress Relief and Calming: Marcasite is renowned for its ability to alleviate stress and anxiety. Its grounding energy promotes a sense of stability and calm, helping to clear the mind and reduce emotional tension. This makes it an excellent companion for meditation and stress management practices.

Mental Clarity: Connected to the root and solar plexus chakras, Marcasite enhances mental clarity and focus. It encourages clear thinking and decision-making, helping individuals to approach challenges with confidence and determination.

Willpower and Strength: Marcasite is a stone of willpower and strength. It supports personal empowerment and resilience, helping individuals to pursue their goals with determination and vigor.

Enhancement of Healing Energies: Known for its ability to amplify healing energies, Marcasite is used to enhance both personal energy and the effectiveness of other healing crystals. It is beneficial in promoting a balanced and harmonious energy flow during healing sessions.

Harmonization and Balance: Marcasite aids in balancing the body's subtle energies. It aligns the chakras and stabilizes emotions, fostering a harmonious internal environment that supports emotional and physical well-being.

Versatile Use in Healing Practices: Utilized in various forms such as raw crystals, jewelry, and meditation tools, Marcasite is a key component in holistic healing practices. It is often used in energy layouts to align and balance the body's energy centers.

Physical Healing Properties

Vitality and Energy: Marcasite is believed to boost physical vitality and energy levels. It helps to invigorate the body, enhancing stamina and overall health.

Detoxification: Marcasite aids in detoxifying the body, supporting liver function and cleansing the system of toxins. This contributes to improved metabolic health and overall well-being.

Immune System: Marcasite is believed to enhance the immune system, helping the body to fight off illnesses more effectively. It

supports the body's natural defenses and promotes overall health and vitality.

Bone and Joint Health: Marcasite supports bone and joint health, helping to strengthen bones and alleviate joint pain. It is beneficial for those dealing with arthritis and other joint-related issues.

Cellular Regeneration: Marcasite supports the body's natural healing processes by promoting cellular regeneration. It aids in the recovery from injuries and illnesses, speeding up the healing process.

Potential Homeopathic Uses

If Marcasite were to be used as a homeopathic remedy, its indications might include:

Psychological Symptoms: Anxiety, emotional stress, and lack of focus. It may also help in cases of emotional instability and lack of willpower.

Physical Symptoms: Detoxification needs, immune system deficiencies, and joint pain.

Behavioral Symptoms: Difficulty in coping with stress, lack of motivation, and a tendency towards emotional imbalance.

Marcasite's homeopathic profile would focus on its ability to ground, protect, and invigorate, making it suitable for addressing conditions related to stress, detoxification, and overall well-being.

Conclusion

Marcasite is a vital crystal in holistic healing, celebrated for its grounding beauty and versatile healing properties. Whether used for stress relief, mental clarity, or as a strengthening talisman, Marcasite serves as a potent aid in achieving physical health and spiritual harmony. Like all alternative practices, these should be considered as complementary to conventional medical treatments.

Chapter Summary

This chapter offers an extensive exploration into the spiritual, emotional, and physical healing properties of unique gemstones. It is designed to provide a holistic understanding of how these gemstones can be utilized within homeopathic and alternative healing practices to promote overall well-being.

At the heart of gemstone homeopathy is the belief in the interconnectedness of the mind, body, and spirit. Each gemstone possesses unique vibrational frequencies that resonate with different aspects of human health. By leveraging these frequencies, practitioners aim to restore balance and harmony, addressing not only physical ailments but also emotional and spiritual imbalances. This approach recognizes that true healing encompasses all dimensions of the self, leading to a more profound and lasting well-being.

Many of the gemstones covered in this chapter are renowned for their ability to enhance spiritual growth and psychic abilities. Stones like Amethyst, Selenite, and Lapis Lazuli are highlighted for their capacity to open the third eye and crown chakras, facilitating deeper meditation, intuition, and spiritual awareness. These gemstones serve as powerful tools for those seeking to deepen their spiritual practice and connect with higher realms of consciousness. The chapter also explores how gemstones like Moldavite and Celestite can assist in astral travel and communication with spirit guides.

Emotional well-being is a significant focus in the Materia Medica. Gemstones such as Rose Quartz, Rhodochrosite, and Lepidolite are celebrated for their soothing and nurturing energies. They help release emotional blockages, heal past traumas, and foster a sense of love, compassion, and inner peace. The chapter provides detailed insights into how these stones can be used to support emotional healing and stability. Additionally, it discusses the role of gemstones like

Moonstone and Amazonite in balancing emotional states and promoting a calm, harmonious disposition.

Protection is a recurring theme throughout the chapter. Gemstones like Black Tourmaline, Hematite, and Smoky Quartz are known for their strong protective properties. They act as energetic shields, safeguarding the user from negative influences, psychic attacks, and electromagnetic pollution. The chapter elaborates on how these stones can be used to create a safe and secure environment for spiritual practices. Furthermore, it examines the protective roles of Obsidian and Shungite, which are particularly effective in grounding and detoxifying energies.

The physical healing attributes of gemstones are thoroughly explored. Stones such as Bloodstone, Carnelian, and Malachite are recognized for their ability to enhance vitality, support the immune system, and promote physical regeneration. The chapter offers comprehensive information on how these gemstones can aid in the recovery from illnesses, alleviate pain, and support overall physical health. It also covers how gemstones like Amber and Chrysocolla can aid in detoxification processes and improve respiratory health, providing a holistic approach to physical wellness.

Detoxification is another critical aspect covered in the Materia Medica. Gemstones like Fluorite, Apatite, and Chrysoprase are noted for their cleansing properties. They assist in purifying the body, mind, and spirit from toxins and negative energies. The chapter provides guidance on using these stones to support detoxification processes and maintain energetic purity. Additionally, it discusses the use of gemstones like Clear Quartz and Citrine in amplifying and focusing cleansing energies, making them indispensable tools in purification rituals.

The chapter emphasizes the importance of chakra balancing in holistic healing. Each gemstone is associated with specific chakras, helping to align and balance the body's energy centers. For example,

Citrine is linked to the solar plexus chakra, promoting confidence and personal power, while Aquamarine resonates with the throat chakra, enhancing communication and self-expression. The Materia Medica offers detailed instructions on using gemstones for chakra healing and alignment, including practical layouts and meditations for optimal energy flow.

Many gemstones are known for their ability to amplify energy, enhancing the effects of other healing practices. Clear Quartz, for instance, is often referred to as the "master healer" for its capacity to amplify the energy of other stones and intentions. The chapter delves into how these amplifying stones can be incorporated into healing rituals to boost their effectiveness. It also explores the synergistic effects of combining gemstones, such as using Amethyst and Rose Quartz together to enhance spiritual and emotional healing.

Each gemstone in the chapter is presented with a detailed homeopathic profile, outlining its psychological, physical, and behavioral indications. This includes descriptions of the symptoms and conditions that the gemstone can address, providing a practical guide for practitioners to select the appropriate stone for their needs. The profiles also highlight the unique energetic signatures of each gemstone, offering a deeper understanding of their healing potential. Special attention is given to rare and powerful gemstones like Phenacite and Larimar, which possess exceptional healing properties.

The chapter concludes with practical advice on incorporating gemstone remedies into daily life. This includes methods for wearing gemstones as jewelry, using them in meditation, placing them in living spaces, and creating gemstone elixirs. The guidance provided ensures that readers can effectively harness the healing properties of gemstones to enhance their well-being. Additionally, the chapter covers advanced techniques such as using gemstone grids for energy work and integrating gemstones into holistic therapies like Reiki and acupuncture.

In summary, the chapter on Materia Medica of gemstone homeopathic remedies is a comprehensive resource that encapsulates the profound healing potential of these unique gemstones. It offers valuable insights into the spiritual, emotional, and physical benefits of gemstones, empowering readers to integrate these powerful tools into their holistic healing practices. This chapter serves as an essential guide for anyone interested in exploring the transformative power of gemstones and their applications in achieving overall well-being.

I hope you enjoyed this book entitled volume two. There are several more volumes on this particular topic which follow.

If you have any questions, please feel free to write me at:

drvictordenispurcell@proton.me

Also by Dr Víctor Denis Purcell

2
Materia Medica of Homeopathic Gemstones

Standalone
Zen and the Way of the Artist
Zen and the Art of Medicine
Zen and the Way of the Artist
The Yoga Book
Zen and the Art of Living and Dying
Zen and the Art of Photography
The Homeopathic Book
das homöopathische buch
El Libro De Homeopatía
Le Livre Homéopathique
The Traveler's Handbook
❖❖❖❖❖❖❖❖❖❖❖
"Architectural and Interior Design Mastery: A Global Perspective"
Medicinal Mushrooms
The New Testament
"Das Neue Testament, 2024"
Новый Завет
Mini Materia Medica

The Receptive Warrior
The God Center
The American Constitution
A Deep Dive Into Death
The Voyager's Odyssey
Mini Materia Medica
Mini Materia Medica
Spiritual Medicine: Materia Medica of Homeopathic Gemstones and Crystals
Spirituelle Medizin: Materia Medica der homöopathischen Edelsteine und Kristalle
Materia Medica of Homeopathic Gemstones
Médecine spirituelle Materia Medica des gemmes et cristaux homéopathiques
Materia Medica of Homeopathic Gemstones
Volume Two: Materia Medica of Homeopathic Gemstones

Also by Victor Denis Purcell

The Voyager's Odyssey
The Big Book of Tarot
Volume Two: Materia Medica of Homeopathic Gemstones

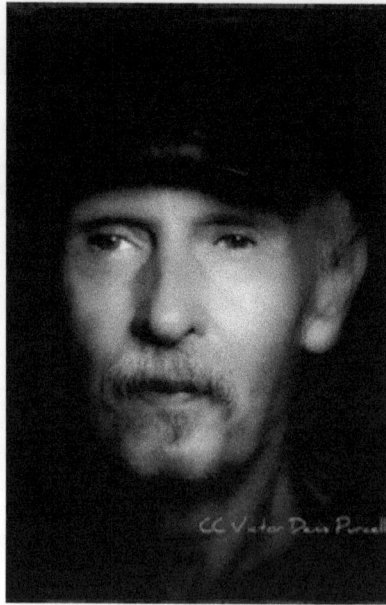

About the Author

Victor Denis Purcell is a certified homeopathic practitioner with a master's degree in educational psychology. With a deep-rooted passion for homeopathic medicine, he has been actively involved in this field since 1982. Over the decades, he has authored numerous books covering a wide range of topics, demonstrating a profound understanding and expertise in homeopathic practices and holistic healing. Through a combination of professional experience and scholarly dedication, Victor Denis Purcell continues to contribute significantly to the advancement and awareness of homeopathic medicine.

Milton Keynes UK
Ingram Content Group UK Ltd.
UKHW030850111124
451035UK00001B/174